DISABILITY, CITIZENSHIP AND COMMUNITY CARE

For Simon and Euan,
with love, thanks and pride

Disability, Citizenship and Community Care

A case for welfare rights?

KIRSTEIN RUMMERY
University of Manchester, UK

Ashgate

Published by
Ashgate Publishing Limited
Gower House
Croft Road
Aldershot
Hampshire GU11 3HR
England

Ashgate Publishing Company
131 Main Street
Burlington, VT 05401-5600 USA

Ashgate website: http://www.ashgate.com

British Library Cataloguing in Publication Data
Rummery, Kirstein
    Disability, citizenship and community care : a case for
    welfare rights?. - (Studies in cash and care)
    1. Handicapped - Services for - England 2. Handicapped - Care
    - England 3. Handicapped - Civil rights - England
    I. Title
    362.4'0483'0942'09049

Library of Congress Control Number: 2001099944

ISBN 0 7546 1757 2

Printed and bound by Athenaeum Press, Ltd.,
Gateshead, Tyne & Wear.

Contents

List of Figures and Tables

Figures

Tables

Preface

This book is a synthesis of theory and research which takes a critical look at the experiences of disabled people accessing and receiving community care services. It has its roots in a Joseph Rowntree funded research project at the University of Birmingham in 1995-1996 which was designed to look at the ways in which disabled people gained access to community care assessments and services (Davis et al, 1997). The bulk of this book is based on analysis of that study data, which comprised of two main sources: ethnographic observations of assessment practice in six social work teams from two local authorities; and in-depth interviews with 46 disabled people and 16 of their family members/friends/supporters who had been through a community care assessment. However, the ideas discussed in this book were developed further after that study, particularly in the light of a Department of Health funded study at the University of Manchester in 1997-1999, designed to look at the experiences of disabled people with complex health and social care needs who used direct payments rather than conventional community care services (Glendinning et al, 2000).

The book develops a citizenship framework of civil and social rights, which is based on seminal work done by Marshall (1992), Plant (1990, 1992), Lister (1995, 1997), Turner (1993a) and Doyal and Gough (1991) among others. It uses that framework to examine the effect of the community care assessment process on the citizenship status of disabled people and their families. For the purposes of this book, 'citizenship status' has three dimensions: the protection or otherwise of a person's civil and social rights (Marshall, 1992); whether or not they are treated as and enabled to act as 'competent members of society' (Turner, 1993a); and whether the process facilitates or prevents disabled people's 'minimally curtailed social participation' (Doyal and Gough, 1991). Chapters one, two and three discuss this framework in more detail.

The ways in which frontline welfare professionals/gatekeepers/ bureaucrats (Klein et al, 1996; Lipsky, 1980) make decisions about who gets access to community care assessments and services, and the impact of these decisions on the citizenship status of disabled people and their families is discussed in chapter four. The ways in which disabled people and their families experience the process of attempting to gain access to assessments and services in the community care process is discussed in chapter five. The remainder of the book is devoted to exploring the effects of the outcome of the community care process on the citizenship status of disabled people and their families, and discussing the relevance of the findings on community care policy. It examines whether there is a case to be made for the adoption of a welfare rights approach to community care for disabled people and their families.

A Quick Note About Terminology

Throughout this book reference is consciously made to 'disabled people and their families'. Whilst this is not terminology that would necessarily be used by the people concerned, it is preferable to any of the alternatives (such as service users, disabled and older people, carers). The people whose experiences form the core of this book had undergone a community care assessment of their needs, and they were mostly people with impairments who were disabled by the social, attitudinal, physical and environmental barriers facing them in society (Oliver, 1990), and whilst their impairments varied they had sufficient commonality of experience to be referred to as disabled. However, for some people their age did make a difference to how they were treated by social services departments, and where this is the case throughout the text they are referred to as 'older disabled people'. The term 'carers' has been largely been avoided, partly because it is problematic for many disabled people (Morris, 1997) who point out that it ignores the fact that many disabled people themselves have caring responsibilities, which is supported by the evidence in the book. The phrase 'disabled people and their families' is therefore used, with one exception. For practitioners carrying out community care assessments there was a clear distinction between the 'disabled person' on the one hand and the 'carer' on the other, and this affected their practices and decision making in several key ways which are discussed in the relevant chapters. Where it is necessary for clarity to highlight these differences (essentially the difference between the person who is nominally the focus of the assessment and the rest of the family) the person *not* the subject of the assessment from the practitioner's point of view is called the 'carer'.

Acknowledgements

Most good social policy research and theory is the result of years of work done by hardworking teams and this book is no exception to that. I am indebted to Ann Davis and Kathryn Ellis who designed the original Joseph Rowntree project and were very generous in allowing me to use the data to develop and test my own theories. I also owe personal and intellectual thanks to colleagues at the National Primary Care Research and Development Centre, University of Manchester who helped me develop my ideas using their data, particularly Caroline Glendinning, Sally Jacobs, Shirley Halliwell and Ruth Young, and to Lisa Tilsley who gave invaluable technical assistance with the manuscript. An intellectual debt is owed to the participants of the various conferences and ESRC seminars at which I discussed the ideas developed in this book.

This book would not have been possible without the involvement of the practitioners who allowed me to observe their practice and the disabled people and their families who took part in interviews. Their insights still inform my work today and I am very grateful. Finally, personal thanks are owed to Simon and Euan Lippmann, without whose co-operation this book would never have left the ground, and Wendy Macdonald and the Bitches on Diets who gave it wings, and Caroline and Adam Povey who babysat and stocked up the fridge when it mattered the most.

1 The Role of Assessments in Community Care for Disabled People in England from 1993

Throughout the 1980s and 1990s many welfare states, particularly those Esping-Anderson characterised as liberal (Esping-Anderson, 1990) such as the UK, found themselves grappling with the issue of rising demand for state-provided benefits and services. At the same time criticism of the way in which the state provided benefits and services began to be voiced by users of those services, such as people with mental health problems, disabled and older people and those with learning disabilities (Oliver and Barnes, 1993; Rogers et al, 1993; Walmsley, 1993; Bell, 1987). The state faced a twin challenge: how to curb rising expenditure while meeting the needs of its citizens. This book is an exploration of the outcome of one state's attempt to tackle those challenges within a fairly narrow context. It focuses on the implementation of one element of community care policy in England in the 1990s: the way in which disabled people attempted to gain access to social care services and support from their local authority social services departments.

In 1990 the British government passed the 1990 NHS and Community Care Act (NHSCCA), a move which represented a substantial shift in policy and practice within the British welfare state. Prior to its implementation access to residential social care services was controlled through the social security benefits system so that disabled people on low incomes could reclaim the cost of board and lodging in residential care from the state. The Griffiths Report (1988) commissioned by the then Conservative administration found that this led to a substantial rise in the numbers of people entering residential care and acted as a disincentive to the development of services aimed at people living in their own homes. Both results were politically unacceptable to a Conservative administration concerned with curbing public expenditure and promoting individual over state responsibility for the provision of social care.

In 1989 the Department of Health issued its blueprint for service change, Caring for People (Department of Health, 1989). It advocated the introduction of a 'quasi-market' (Le Grand and Bartlett, 1993) in social care, designating local authority social services departments as those responsible for purchasing residential and domiciliary care services for disabled and older people from a mixed market of statutory and private sector providers. It also set up the functions of assessment and care management as the 'cornerstone' of its new policy (Department of Health, 1990: 3).

The Cornerstone of Community Care

As far as the Conservative administration and the Griffiths Report was concerned, the rise in public expenditure on residential care services which resulted from the social security system rules (Laing, 1993) needed to be addressed. The proposed solutions set out in the 1989 White Paper included the driving principle that the provision of services to disabled and older people should be *needs-led* rather than based on income. Local authority social services departments were therefore firstly allocated the responsibility for assessing the needs of individual disabled and older people who appeared to need their services (s47 NHSCCA). Secondly, they became responsible for the process of care management, whereby a care manager put together a package of services from a variety of providers to meet that individual's needs, a process developed following innovative pilots in Kent, Gateshead and Darlington (see for example Challis et al, 1995).

The NHSCCA did differ in some of its key policy objectives from the original 1988 Griffiths Report (Means and Smith, 1994) but the policy of using assessment and care management as a tool to foster needs-led services remained intact. It was recognised that the implementation of many of the provisions of the 1990 Act would be difficult for local authorities and it was not until 1993 that the act was fully implemented in England and Wales.

Positioning the responsibility for assessment and care management with local authority social services departments had several implications for the way in which disabled and older people gained access to residential and domiciliary social care services. Firstly, notwithstanding the criticisms of residential services (Townsend, 1962; Goffman, 1961) not least those coming from disabled people themselves (Morris, 1993b; Brisenden, 1985;

UPIAS, 1976) the introduction of assessment was the introduction of an additional level of gatekeeping and removed from disabled people the 'right' to access such care (Glendinning, 1991). Secondly, it explicitly vested in social services employees (rather than disabled people themselves) the power and discretion to make potentially significant decisions about who should be allowed to access which services. Disabled citizens would have to go through an 'assessment' undertaken by social services before they could access residential or domiciliary care services. Thirdly, it gave local authorities the discretion to design and implement their own assessment and care management systems, which, because local authorities in England and Wales are funded partly through local taxation, meant that spending and service priorities, and hence assessment and care management systems, varied considerably across the country (Audit Commission, 1996).

Disabled Citizens

If assessment and care management were the 'cornerstone' of community care policy (Deartment of Health, 1989) and practice, what building or structure were they meant to be supporting? Chapter three discusses in some depth the conflicting aims and objectives inherent in the 1990 community care changes, particularly how these conflicts were played out within the context of assessment policy and practice. As the changes were implemented it became increasingly clear that frontline practitioners carrying out assessments were having to 'square the circle' of these conflicts within their daily practice (Ellis, 1993). The aims and objectives of community care policy therefore have an impact on the way in which disabled people can access residential and domiciliary care services. The cornerstone appeared to be designed to support several structures at the same time, most notably the push to curb expenditure and to encourage the provision of informal family support rather than statutory services.

This book is concerned with the citizenship status of disabled people and the way in which statutory processes (in this case the way in which disabled people access a community care assessment and thus services) can affect this status. The citizenship framework used throughout this book will be discussed in more depth in chapter two. In summary it is developed from Marshall's seminal essay (Marshall, 1992) which argued that citizenship was made up of political, civil and social rights granted to individuals to both ameliorate the power of the state and make income inequalities and class distinctions less important. Turner (1993a) maintained that people were defined as being citizens if they were considered to be 'competent members of society' and that the 'various social arrangements whereby...benefits are distributed to different sectors of society' (Turner, 1993a: 2-3) was of prime concern to people's citizenship status. Within community care policy post 1990 it is the assessment process which is designed to distribute the 'benefits' of social care services to disabled people. This book examines the assessment process from a citizenship perspective and ask whether it protects or enhances, or acts as a barrier to disabled people's status as 'competent members of society', how it affects their civil and social rights, and whether it enables or prevents people from participating in society.

However, protecting or enhancing the citizenship status of disabled people was never one of the explicit or implicit aims of community care policy. No reference is made throughout the Griffiths Report, White Paper or legislation to citizenship, rights or any other key terms associated with citizenship, although phrases such as 'promoting choice and independence' 'involving users' and so on do appear throughout the policy and practice recommendations (Department of Health, 1989; SSI/SSWG, 1991). The 1990 community care changes were drafted with the stated intention of improving the lives of those who received social care services, but such intentions were not necessarily constructed within a citizenship framework. Alongside the structural changes to social care services and the procedural changes to the way in which people accessed those services a change to the ethos and driving values of social services departments was intended to take place. Disabled people were to be recast in the role of 'consumers' of services, experiencing 'empowerment' through the introduction of market mechanisms into social care services and increased independence through needs-led, domiciliary-based services.

Chapter three will discuss the limitations of this marketised approach in empowering the consumers of social care services. However, it is not the aim of this book to examine the success or failure of the 1990 community care changes to create consumerist improvements for users of social care services. There have been many studies which have focused on the limitations of choice offered to users by the introduction of consumerist elements to social care (see for example Wistow et al, 1996; Baldock and Ungerson, 1993; Hardy et al, 1999; Barnes and Prior, 1995). There have also been studies which focus on the outcome of community care policy which have taken an analysis closer to that used in this book: i.e. the extent to which services have offered users independence and control (see for example Morris, 1993a, 1993b).

Few studies have adopted an explicit citizenship framework to analyse the impact of the community care changes. In part this is because the language and normative core of the policy had an explicitly consumerist rather than citizenship focus (Bynoe, 1996). It is also rarer to see an analysis that is explicitly citizenship centred within a political system that does not have a written constitution i.e. where the relationship between individuals and the state is subject to rules laid down in statutory and common law rather than one in which there is an explicit single document delineating that relationship. This is perhaps why disabled people themselves have been slower to model themselves as citizens accessing rights than, for example, in the United States (Driedger, 1989) where campaigns for income and services for disabled people have been linked to civil rights and anti discrimination campaigns. Where disabled people have attempted to use the language of rights to highlight shortcomings in community care provision this has tended to backfire, as in the high profile Gloucestershire ruling where it was decided that social services departments had a duty to take resources into account when assessing the needs of disabled people, reaffirming that disabled people do not have an automatic right to access social care services (Drewett, 1999).

Nevertheless, simply because disabled people do not have a recognisable automatic right to access services does not mean that they do not have 'rights' within the assessment process, nor that the implementation of the 1990 community care changes does not have any bearing on their citizenship status. One of the most important pre-existing rights that the NHSCCA upheld was the right (granted under the 1986 Disabled Persons (Services, Consultation, Representation) Act) for disabled people to access an assessment of their needs. In fact, s47 of the NHSCCA actually extended the duty on social services departments to assess the needs of anyone appearing to need their services, not just disabled people. Moreover, as will become clear in chapter two, within a Marshallian approach to citizenship it is entirely consistent that access to resources should be rationed by welfare professionals while at the same time individual citizens have the 'right' to access resources to meet their needs - the fact that it is contingent on the availability of resources does not make it not a 'right'.

Citizenship and Community Care: The Aims of This Book

This book therefore attempts to address the balance by using an explicit citizenship framework to critically analyse the impact of the NHSCCA on the lives of disabled people. It examines the effect of the assessment process on the citizenship status of disabled people by asking whether their civil and social rights are threatened or protected by it. How do frontline welfare professionals decide who gets access to an assessment and social care services, and how do these decisions affect the social participation or exclusion of disabled people and their families? How do disabled people and their families experience attempts to access an assessment, and then within the assessment to negotiate their needs and access to services and support to meet those needs? What effects does the outcome of the assessment process (i.e. the services, equipment and support - or lack of it - received) have on the social participation or exclusion of disabled people and their families? And what might the impact of an explicitly citizen-friendly community care policy - one based on welfare rights - be on social services departments, disabled people and their families?

2 Social Policy, Rights and Citizenship

Since Marshall's seminal essay on the theme (Marshall, 1992), the nature of citizenship has pre-occupied social policy analysts. In particular, Marshall's concept of social citizenship has been revisited by academics in response to the critique of the welfare state from the 'New Right'. This chapter will briefly outline some of the current debates on social citizenship and examine whether it is a useful theoretical tool to understand disabled people's relationships with social services departments as the latter undertake the assessment and care management tasks discussed in the previous chapter.

Social Citizenship

The basic definition of citizenship used in this book, which encompasses social citizenship, stems from Turner's analysis of the relationship between individuals, their rights and entitlements, and the policies and practices which dictate whether and how individuals can claim those rights and entitlements (Turner, 1990, 1993a, 1993b). He outlines his theory of citizenship thus:

> Citizenship may be defined as that set of practices (juridical, political, economic and cultural) which define a person as a competent member of society, and which as a consequence shape the flow of resources to persons and social groups...Citizenship is concerned with (a) the content of social rights and obligations; (b) with the form or type of such obligations and rights; (c) with the social forces that produces such practices; and finally (d) with the various social arrangements whereby such benefits are distributed to different sectors of society (Turner, 1993a: 2-3).

Turner's formulation is a development of ideas first discussed by Marshall in his seminal 1950 essay Citizenship and Social Class (Marshall, 1992). Marshall saw the concept of citizenship as part of the evolution of nation states. The nineteenth century (in Western Europe) saw citizenship being separated into political and civil citizenship, with the introduction of the franchise to a wider range of the population than the landed gentry. However, neither political nor civil citizenship were available universally until the twentieth century.

The evolution of social citizenship is, according to Marshall, a more recent phenomenon. Since the Elizabethan Poor Law, social rights have been detached from the status of citizenship. In fact, the protection of charity and a notion of social rights was only relevant for those excluded from full citizenship, such as women, children and those living in poverty. It is only with the development of a 'universal' welfare state that the concept of social citizenship acquires any real meaning, as it is only the welfare state which gives citizens access to social rights which do not compromise their citizenship.

For Marshall, 'citizenship is a status bestowed on those who are full members of a community' (Marshall, 1992: 18). He failed, however, to discuss fully what he meant by 'full members' and 'community', concepts which will be discussed further below. Full citizenship was not, he argued, limited by the inequalities of social class. Indeed, the function of the social rights bestowed by the welfare state, and this full social citizenship, was meant to undermine the inequalities inherent in the class system. Barbalet has argued that:

> the issue of who can practice citizenship and on what terms is not only a matter of the legal scope of citizenship and the formal nature of the rights entailed in it. It is also a matter of the non-political capacities of citizens which derive from the social resources they command and to which they have access (Barbalet, 1988: 1).

The gaining of social rights is therefore vital for any individual or group claiming the status of citizenship.

The function of social rights was not, however, to equalise income and so remove class inequalities. Marshall maintained that 'equality of status is more important than equality of income' (Marshall, 1992: 33). The fact that each citizen had equal 'claim rights' (rights to access resources) against the welfare state, depending on need, was intended to create a universal citizenship while being reconciled to an unequal society. Turner points out that this meant the institute of citizenship 'functioned to ameliorate the condition of the working class without transforming the entire property system' (Turner, 1993b: 177).

Barbalet summarises Marshall's thinking thus: 'Advances in the form of citizenship are likely to leave class structures intact, although class loyalty and class resentment may be affected by the removal of particular disadvantages' (Barbalet, 1988: 5). Dahrendorf has asserted that 'whatever citizenship does to social class, it does not eliminate either inequality or conflict. It changes their quality' (Dahrendorf, 1996: 42). This suggests that Marshall may have been disingenuous in stressing the way that citizenship rights do not substantially alter class relations. While the welfare state in the UK has failed to substantially attack inequalities and poverty, it has contributed to the dramatic social changes which have in turn affected social, political and civil structures over the last fifty years (Lister, 1990; Culpitt, 1992). Nevertheless, Marshall was very clear that his concept of social rights did not necessarily encompass the right to any particular benefits or services.

Marshall illustrated his thesis by pointing out that every citizen had the right to be registered with a doctor. However, there is no accompanying right to any medical treatment or services - no citizen is guaranteed this his ailments will be properly cared for or that he will receive any particular treatments (I am using the male pronoun advisedly in this section, as Marshall did not include any concept of gendered citizenship in his analysis). Nevertheless, the formation of the National Health Service was founded on the principle that each citizen had to the right to access health care according to their needs, although it did not give citizens guaranteed access to any particular services. Therefore, the main social rights of citizens were the rights to equality of opportunity, rather than equality of outcomes.

The formulation of the concept of social rights included a concept of the duties and obligations accompanying those rights. Marshall pointed out that 'if citizenship is invoked in the name of rights, the corresponding duties of citizenship cannot be ignored' (Marshall, 1992: 41). Thus political citizenship is complemented by the duty to engage in the political process (hence the legal duty, in the UK, for citizens to ensure that their names are on the electoral role). Civil citizenship comes with various duties not to infringe the civil code (which is why prisoners are not entitled to vote). Similarly, social citizenship is complemented by social duties, which, within the context of the UK welfare state, has tended to mean the duty to work (and originally meant engaging in public, paid work rather than unpaid, private work). The concept of social duties is also further discussed below.

The concept of social citizenship has recently come under sustained attack from both the 'New Right' (such as policy commentators from the Adam Smith Institute, among others) and the 'New Left' (for example, the Institute for Public Policy Research). The remainder of this chapter will be used to outline those attacks, and examine whether the concept of social citizenship can be reclaimed, or reconstituted to provide a useful tool for analysis of the experiences of disabled citizens approaching social services departments for help, advice or services - an approach which is constituted by the latter as an approach for an 'assessment of needs'.

The 'Myth' Of Social Citizenship

Critics of Marshall's theory of social citizenship and the evolution of social rights as part of society's evolution towards full civilisation have come mainly from right-wing and liberal academics. Their opposition to social citizenship is located within two broad arguments. The first concentrates on social rights as 'positive' rights which require some redistribution of resources, as distinct from 'negative' political and civil rights. The second focuses on the way in which social rights interfere with the workings of the market, particularly the importance of the individual as a free agent within the market.

'Positive' Versus 'Negative' Rights

The 'New Right' liberals who dispute the existence of social citizenship claim that social rights are fundamentally different from political and civil rights (Hayek, 1960; Friedman, 1962; Barry, 1987). As Marshall himself asserted, the claim to any rights is meaningless without a corresponding acknowledgement of the duties that accompany them. The liberal critique of social rights rests on their claim that the duties accompanying social rights are fundamentally different from the duties accompanying political and civil rights.

Political and civil duties are essentially negative duties of non-interference in another's liberties. Plant summarises this argument thus:

> The right to life is the right to be free from being killed, the
> right to freedom of speech is the right to speak and not be
> silenced, the rights to physical integrity and security are rights
> to be free from assault, rape and coercion of various sorts.

> Because these are rights to be free from interference of specific types, the corresponding duties on the part of fellow citizens, government and social agencies are to abstain from killing, interfering, raping, coercing and so forth. The right to life is not the positive right to the means to life (Plant, 1992: 18).

Civil and political duties are essentially negative - duties not to do things - which therefore do not carry any cost implications (financial or otherwise) for the bearer of the duty. It costs me nothing not to kill or harm another person, nor to not prevent them from speaking. Civil and political rights are therefore meaningful because they can always be respected without any burden on the individual, group or society respecting those rights. Hayek (1960) maintained that the duty *not* to coerce people to do things is distinct from giving people the ability to actually do them, which would impose a financial or physical cost on those individuals or groups granting the ability.

Social rights, on the other hand, are positive rights to things that entail a positive duty to provide the resources to supply those things. As such, they rely on the concept of human need - people must have needs, otherwise social rights would be unnecessary (Doyal and Gough, 1991). However, because meeting those needs entails resource implications, it follows that access to social rights must be rationed and that social rights are therefore by definition always limited. There is no consensus on how this rationing should take place, and so an element of moral judgement in balancing the needs of one individual or group against another (Burkitt and Davey, 1984). This renders social rights in the eyes of liberals meaningless (Barry, 1987). To make any rights meaningful they must have clear limits and always be capable of being discharged (Plant, 1992) and not simply be a political interpretation of need (Fraser, 1989).

Lonely Citizens, the Market and the Welfare State

The second main theme running through the liberal critique of social rights and social citizenship is that social rights interfere with the operation of the market. They do so firstly because they involve the commitment and redistribution of resources according to need rather than according to market worth, and secondly because they interfere with individual freedoms.

The liberal challenge presumes that people are essentially individualistic (Ignatieff, 1984). Acting as free agents, they are what Culpitt calls 'lonely citizens' (Culpitt, 1992: 6). As such, they can comply only with the 'negative' duties of civil and political citizenship without coercion. Any 'positive' duties would require coercion on an individualistic agent, and it makes no sense for individuals to have to be coerced into being citizens. Moreover, in order for the market to function fully, it is necessary for agents to be individualistic, to be able to compete and sell their labour at the market price.

The ethics of social redistribution are therefore questionable for liberals. Why should a lonely citizen or individualistic agent feel an obligation to provide for those less well off? The welfare state has thus been characterised as a 'coercive bargain between strangers which abridge(s) the liberties of both rich and poor while infantilising the poor' (Ignatieff, 1989: 63). The welfare state, in trying to effect social redistribution, has undermined the market and led to the dependency of certain groups of people, notably the poor (Murray, 1990). Furthermore, the liberal argument hinges on the assertion that the welfare state has done little towards creating social justice and meaningful social rights, and has substantially undermined the market's efforts to create individual social justice (Lane, 1987).

The welfare state, as the conduit for social redistribution, is also viewed as cumbersome, ineffective, bound by bureaucracy and unresponsive to individual needs (Weddell, 1986). Due to 'perverse incentives' that mean that their success is measured according to how protected and powerful their own agency becomes under their management, public sector managers are more concerned with building their 'empires' than in effectively meeting need (Bennett and Johnson, 1980). The welfare state has become enmeshed in its own legitimacy and performance, and has failed to deliver social justice (Drucker, 1969). Agents of the welfare state have become 'administrators without law', operating with a high degree of discretion with the minimum of accountability (Friedman, 1981). Therefore, claiming social rights against the state does not confer social citizenship, as the rights are not universal and depend upon this discretion.

This critique of the welfare state is not limited to the New Right - other writers have noted the malign effects of government agencies (Turner, 1986) and their unresponsiveness to meeting need (Taylor-Gooby, 1985; Gronbjerg, 1983). However, within liberal policy, this view of the welfare state has led to the introduction of privatisation and quasi-markets in the delivery of social welfare (LeGrand and Robinson, 1984; Bosanquet, 1983), in an effort to make the welfare state more effective at responding to needs. Nevertheless, any restructuring in the delivery of social welfare tends to lead to a reduction in access to services (Lipsky, 1980), and the effect of the introduction of quasi-markets has been, in part, a sustained erosion of universal access to services resulting in the welfare state playing a residual role in the provision of social services (Glendinning, 1993).

In an effort to move away from the concept of the lonely citizen as an individual agent, liberal theorists have concentrated on the idea of the 'active citizen' (Mead, 1986). This is an idea that found favour with the previous Conservative government in the UK (Lister, 1990). The 'active citizen' is one who discharges his or her obligations to society through working, paying taxes and carrying out voluntary work - in other words, the concept of the active citizen focuses clearly on individual duties, and shifts the focus away from individual rights against the state. In a curious about turn, the New Right has shifted from claiming that social rights are a nonsense because of the lack of consensus on what constitutes needs, to claiming the moral superiority of giving over receiving welfare (Lister, 1990, Selbourne, 1994).

Universal Social Citizenship?

The New Right's attack on social citizenship has, in its turn, attracted sustained criticism from 'New Left' writers who have argued that the liberal position is based on a series of unsustainable assumptions (Dahrendorf, 1988; Turner, 1990; Roche, 1992; Lister, 1990). One of the main critiques has been the false nature of the 'negative' versus 'positive' rights divide, which is discussed below. However, the New Left are not uncritical of either Marshall's concept of universal social citizenship, nor the welfare state itself, pointing out that both operate oppressively towards some groups.

'Negative' Versus 'Positive' Rights

Raymond Plant has provided one of the most comprehensive attacks on the ideological suppositions of the New Right (Plant, 1992, 1988, 1990). He points out that the distinction between 'negative' civil and political rights, and 'positive' social rights is a fallacy. Rights are distinguished from other claims in that they are enforceable, and enforcing rights, whether it be through the use of laws, police forces or armies, entails a significant cost.

Echoing Marshall's example of the right to access a doctor not entailing the right to access any particular treatment, Plant points out that 'members of the public have no legally enforceable right to particular policing services in relation to any public incident' (Plant, 1992: 22). He argues that Hayek's distinction between freedom and ability is equally tenuous:

What makes liberty valuable is that we are enabled to do things with the space within which we are not coerced by others. However, if it is this ability which makes freedom valuable then it could be argued that there is a conceptual link between freedom and ability; it is our ability to do things that makes freedom worth struggling for (Plant, 1990: 14).

In other words, because civil and political rights need enforcing, they cannot be said to be negative rights. Freedom from coercion is only meaningful if gaining it means gaining the ability to do something - therefore all 'negative' rights are essentially 'positive' rights. Citizenship, if it is a status worth struggling for, must entail positive gains. The sometimes fatal struggles for citizenship experienced by suffragettes at the beginning of the twentieth century, and the ongoing struggles for citizenship experienced by ethnic minorities and aboriginal groups show that citizenship is still considered worth struggling for (Turner, 1990; Cass, 1994).

The liberal argument that the existence of 'positive' social rights is a fallacy because of the lack of consensus on what constitutes need has also been criticised. There are various mechanisms that can be deployed to reach a consensus within society on what constitutes need, from democratic participation and political negotiation allowing communities to define their own needs (Beresford and Croft, 1993), to particular mechanisms allowing small groups of people to decide on priorities and needs in particular situations, such as citizen's juries within health purchasing (Cooper et al, 1995). While these may be process-oriented, they are in substance not so different from mechanisms that have historically been used to decide who should have access to 'negative' political and civil rights, such as property ownership, membership of the militia, residence, gender, race and religion (Rees, 1996). There has always been a lack of consensus over who should have access to both 'negative' AND 'positive' rights. The example of the lack of human rights experienced by people with mental health problems highlights that this lack of consensus continues (Rogers and Pilgrim, 1989; Bell, 1987).

The Market and Consumerism

One of the underpinning themes of the New Right's critique of social citizenship is that it is an ineffective way of empowering the beneficiaries of the welfare state. They argue that service users have been disempowered by the inefficiency of the welfare state at responding to need (Weddell,

1986), and that the only way to tackle this is to marketise the welfare state to make it more responsive to need (Burkitt and Davey, 1984). This has resulted in the UK with policy moves to introduce 'quasi-markets' into the welfare state, particularly into the delivery of health and social care (Bosanquet, 1983; LeGrand and Bartlett, 1993).

Certain key concepts underpin the effort, through marketisation, to make the welfare state more responsive to need. They include *participation, consultation, choice* and *empowerment. Participation* encompasses the efforts made to involve the end-users of services in decisions about services, including both 'macro-involvement' in service development and 'micro-involvement' in negotiating individuals' access to services (Croft and Beresford, 1990). *Consultation* is, arguably, at the lower end of user involvement, as its focus is on less than full participation in decisions about services (Barnes, 1999). *Choice* and *empowerment* are indelibly linked in a marketised welfare state, as it is through exercising choice in the welfare service 'market' that the end-user (who will be conceived as a 'consumer' within a marketised system) will be empowered - that is, becoming what Turner calls 'competent members of society' (Turner, 1993a: 2).

However, there are limits to how far markets can empower the end-users of services, for several reasons. Firstly, it has not been possible (or politically desirable) to make the welfare state act as a 'real' market. Competition between providers has not been between providers operating with the same profit-motives or for the same measurable 'gains' to consumers. In the example of community care chosen by the author to illustrate the relationship between citizens and the state, the consumers within this 'quasi-market' are not the end-users of services whose needs the market is meant to meet, but the health and social care purchasers who buy services on their behalf (Barnes, 1997, 1999). The end-users have limited power to change the markets as they have limited power to chose their services, or opt-out of services in the face of little alternative provision. In some cases, the concept of choice in welfare provision is meaningless because end-users are given little or no choice in whether or not they receive services - such as those who compulsorily admitted for mental health 'treatment' (Rogers and Pilgrim, 1989; Bell, 1987) or those who cannot access services they need because they are not available, are considered too expensive or because they do not have the status required to access services (such as residency). The concept of consumers being empowered through exercising choice in the welfare market is therefore a fallacy.

Secondly, the purchasers making the buying decisions in social care are professionals with their own interests and tendencies toward protectionism (Clarke and Newman, 1997). While policy makers have attempted to address this by introducing a user-focused managerialism into health and social care purchasing (NHSME, 1992), this in itself does not empower the end-users of services as managers focus on monitoring contracts to meet specification which they, not the end-users, have set (Walsh, 1995). In fact, managerialism has served to sustain professionals' power in the relationship between users and purchasers of welfare services because it has strengthened the emphasis on effective budgeting and consequently lessened the emphasis on ascertaining need (Ellis, 1993), although this emphasis arguably does not meet professionals' needs any better than those of end-users.

Therefore aiming to empower individuals by recreating their image in the welfare state as consumers is a strategy bound to meet with limited success. The mechanics of such a strategy has resulted, in British social policy, in a focus on changing the relationships between service providers and purchasers, rather than between service providers and users (Barnes and Walker, 1996). Consumerism can only facilitate a two-party relationship, that between a purchaser and (potential) provider of goods or services. The fact that there can be more than one potential provider does not undermine the bipartisan nature of the consumerist relationship. It cannot operate to empower either service users or carers because they do not have 'purchasing power' within the relationship.

The consumerist discourse is therefore in opposition to a discourse in social policy which focuses on citizenship and rights, as the latter is concerned not with the relationships between purchasers and providers within the 'internal market' of the welfare state, but with the relationship between the individual and the state. Within a consumerist community care policy this relationship is therefore between the service user (the 'quasi consumer') and the service purchaser (the state). There is no room in the relationship for the 'third party' in community care - service providers, either paid or unpaid carers (Biggs, 1994). However, it is the multiple relationships between the purchasers, providers and recipients of care which characterises community care, rather than the one-to-one relationship that can be enhanced by the introduction of quasi-markets (Finch, 1989). Efforts to address this limitation to consumerism have been made within British social policy by the introduction of direct payments to certain categories of service users, to enable them to purchase their own care. Guidance on direct payments suggests that users have to undergo the same assessments as they would if they were receiving services purchased on their behalf, so an element of the tripartite purchaser/provider/user relationship remains (Department of Health, 1999). However, as will be discussed within chapter six, giving disabled people cash instead of services does enable them to exercise some degree of choice and control over the support they receive, as compared to receiving traditional services. There does appear to be a limited element of consumerism that can work to empower disabled people.

However, the consumerist discourse within the welfare state has therefore rightly been criticised as failing to empower either individual end users of services, or groups of people who should, theoretically, be empowered by Marshall's social rights. The welfare state itself has also been criticised by those on the 'New Left' as failing to deliver Marshall's promised social citizenship, particularly as it has failed to deliver universal social citizenship.

The 'Myth' of the Universal Welfare State

Critics on both the 'New Right' and the 'New Left' have pointed out that the welfare state is not a morally neutral mechanism delivering public good (Friedman, 1981; Ignatieff, 1984; Culpitt, 1992). The middle classes arguably benefit disproportionately from the universal elements of welfare provision, such as the NHS and the education system (Le Grand, 1982) whilst those elements of the welfare state that are means tested, such as income replacement benefits and social care, end up both stigmatising those who access them, and incorporating proportionately higher costs for the middle classes (Goodin and LeGrand, 1987; Murray, 1990). The welfare state has not eradicated poverty (Townsend, 1979), although Marshall's defence of social citizenship did point out that it would never equalise income, only ameliorate the effects of unequal income and thus remove inter-class tension (Barbalet, 1993).

One key issue that Marshall failed to address was that social divisions other than class and income are responsible for the unequal access to full political, civil and social citizenship experienced by the British population. Given that, at the time he delivered his lecture, French women had only just achieved universal suffrage, and some Swiss women were to wait 29 years before being able to vote in canton elections, his uncritical conceptualisation of social citizenship evolving from full political and civil citizenship masked the gendered nature of citizenship (Walby, 1994). The absence of a focus on women's needs in the evolution of the welfare state has had clear repercussions for women's citizenship. Lister points out that:

> The interplay between social and political citizenship has been key in the development of women's position as citizens in the twentieth century. The nature of the social rights that have emerged has, in part, been a reflection of the extent to which

women have been involved politically in their construction (Lister, 1995: 7).

Marshall's theory of citizenship was based on the idea that social citizenship evolved from political and civil citizenship, as citizenship became a status less associated with membership of a city-state and more with membership of a nation-state (Turner, 1990). However, evidence from the evolution of women's citizenship, particularly in the former Communist countries, would suggest that it is possible for elements of social citizenship to preclude full civil and political citizenship (Einhorn, 1993). This argument is echoed by Scandinavian feminist writers, who point out that even if a welfare state guarantees women full access to social rights, it does not guarantee women full political and civil citizenship (Hernes, 1987).

Women's restricted access to full civil and political citizenship, as characterised by their underrepresentation in 'public' political activity, is mirrored by their overrepresentation in 'private' community activity. This has led to the development two strands of debate on women's citizenship. The first seeks to reclaim the concept of 'active' citizenship, repositing it as one in which women's participation in the collective live of the community (mainly through unpaid care for children, spouses and relatives) is accorded the same citizenship status as is at present accorded to participation in public political and civil activity (such as undertaking paid work or engaging in the democratic process of a nation-state) (Mouffe, 1992; Finch, 1985; Finch and Groves, 1980; Pateman, 1992). The second is, to a certain extent, in opposition to the first, as it stresses the importance of women accessing full civil and political citizenship by 'active engagement in the public world' (Dietz, 1987: 15), through becoming radical, democratic political beings. However, as Lister argues, 'a rounded and fruitful theorisation of citizenship...has to embrace both individual rights (and, in particular, social rights) and political participation and has also to analyse the relationship between the two' (Lister, 1995: 7).

Formulating a theory to explain women's citizenship has other pitfalls, as it does not take account of the fact that the category 'woman' is contestable. The idea that there is anything like a universal claim to citizenship that is shared by all women is contested by black women (hooks, 1982), lesbian women (Kitzinger, 1987) and disabled women (Morris, 1991), among others. Women may have particular citizenship claims, but different categories of women will have different categories of claims. However, it is possible to work with a concept of difference and yet maintain an idea of universal social citizenship. Firstly, the welfare state can be said to operate in a sufficiently gendered way that a gendered notion of citizenship does have meaning (Walby, 1994; Lister, 1995, 1997). Secondly, women's difference does not obviate their claim to equal access to citizenship - the opposite of equal access is unequal access, not difference.

Similar arguments could be made when examining disabled people's access to social citizenship. On the front of one of the key texts from the disabled people's movement, Oliver's *The Politics of Disablement*, there is a picture of a young man in a wheelchair outside a polling station, unable to enter the building and cast his vote because the entrance to the building is via a flight of steps. It is a powerful image that encapsulates disabled people's exclusion from full civil and political citizenship. Yet different disabled people, with different impairments, experience that exclusion in different ways - the picture would have made no sense if the young man had had epilepsy, been deaf or had any other impairments unrelated to stairclimbing. This 'difference' does not change the fact that 'disabled people', as a universal category, are excluded from full citizenship. Similar points have been made with regards to race and age (Williams, 1989).

The disabled people's movement's response to the way the state actively facilitates disabled people's exclusion from full citizenship has focused around the 'social model of disability'. This model seeks to explain how people with impairments are 'disabled' by the cultural, environmental and physical barriers that society creates, rather than by their own impairments. Oliver traces these barriers as having developed in Western society at the same time as capitalism (Oliver, 1990). The social model has its limitations in explaining disabled people's exclusion from full participation in society. By concentrating on disabled people's relationship to the state through a materialist analysis of their role in the capitalist process (for example how disabled people have been excluded from paid work by the industrial revolution), the social model falls into the same trap as the New Right - its proponents view citizenship simply in terms of access to the political and civil benefits of work. In order to explain disabled people's exclusion from full participation in society, it is necessary to examine whether or not they are excluded from accessing full social citizenship.

The welfare state has attracted criticism from other users of its services, particularly disabled people (Barnes, 1991) and people with mental health problems (Bell, 1987; Rogers and Pilgrim, 1989), who have experienced the effects of social policies ostensibly designed to meet Marshall's description of social rights and social citizenship. They point out that the welfare state can operate at best in a bureaucratic, professionally driven way, and at worst can severely abuse and brutalise the end users of services. The self-depiction of mental health service users as 'survivors' of the psychiatric system is a clear indication that access to social services is not always experienced in terms of accessing full social citizenship, and that the welfare state can in fact exclude end users of its services from citizenship.

Responses to Unequal Citizenship

The Left's solution to the unequal way in which different individuals access full citizenship is to focus on increasing the democratic accountability of all the branches of the state, including the welfare state. One recent example of this in the UK is the move towards decentralised parliaments in Scotland and Wales. The limitations of this approach are that increasing democratic accountability and participation relies on groups of individuals having what Plant calls 'a politics of common identity' (Plant, 1990: 4). Within social classes and other social divisions, it is clear from the feminist debate on difference that there is little evidence that social classes or divisions have that kind of identity within a pluralistic society. Individuals within modern British society can be said to have a 'polyhedra' of identities and allegiances which do not lend themselves easily to sustaining a common group identity (Williams, 1989). A further limitation to this approach is that the political process is characterised by competing interest groups which do not have compatible aims, and that competing claims to political representation would either have to measured against a moral framework, or a consensus reached that would simply serve the lowest common denominator of interests.

The New Right's solution is to reformulate the relationship between individuals and the state as a marketised, consumerist relationship. One example of this is the profusion of citizen's charters produced by the Conservative government in the UK in the 1990s, which aimed to reposition end users of welfare state services as customers with the right to expect the levels of services in the public sector which consumers enjoy in the private sector (Bynoe, 1996). The limits of this approach have been discussed above. The way forward from these competing theories of the crisis of the welfare state is to reclaim the concept of social citizenship for end users of its services.

Reclaiming Social Citizenship

If end users of the welfare state are to achieve a status that goes beyond being either a consumer, or democratic participant, in the welfare state, then the concept of social citizenship has to be reclaimed. A welfare system whereby individuals can assert claim rights against the state, rather than being consumers within a quasi-market place, clients within a professional/bureaucratic relationship, or consulted democratic agents, is the key to establishing universal access to social citizenship. The test of how any welfare benefit or service operates should therefore be whether or not it enables the recipients of that benefit or service to be empowered as citizens - to be 'competent members of society' (Turner, 1993a), to be able to exercise choices about the way in which they discharge their responsibilities and duties to society as well as participate actively as a member of society. As such, it is necessary to test the various practices of the welfare state to establish the relationship between individuals, their social rights, and the state. Being able to attain citizenship as described above is dependent in part on individuals being able to assert civil and social rights against the state.

In the context of this book, I intend to examine the various dimensions of citizenship from the perspective of disabled people attempting to gain access to social rights to enable them to participate in society as fully competent members of that society. The relationship between the Marshallian notion of civil and social rights and the process of gaining access to social rights is explored more fully in the next chapter, and the role that the community care assessment plays in the process in practice is discussed in chapter four. Subsequent chapters will develop the citizenship framework more fully to explain the decisions taken by practitioners about who should access civil and social rights, and the consequences of those decisions for the citizenship status of disabled people and their families. However, before we move on to developing and applying the citizenship framework to disabled people and their families as they go through the process of community care assessments, there are some problems with the concept of social rights that need to be addressed.

Social Rights - a Right to Welfare?

Social rights are problematic as a philosophical and legal concept, as they are essentially claim rights to income or services against a finite supply. A right to something is an enforceable choice to that thing, but theories of rights which concentrate on rights as enforceable choices are inadequate at explaining or supporting rights that citizens who cannot enforce them themselves (such as frail older people) have against the state (Goodin and

Gibson, 1997). This book has already discussed the false distinction between negative and positive rights by pointing out that both types of rights entail cost, and could therefore be conceptualised as positive rights (Plant, 1990). Nevertheless, as Marshall points out, citizens cannot meaningfully assert the right to any services, so where does that leave the concept of social citizenship?

In order to reclaim social citizenship as a useful concept for disabled people attempting to assert their 'right' to those services which would give them access to social citizenship, they must be able to enforce those rights against the state. Alcock makes this argument in relation to what he calls 'welfare rights':

> Welfare rights challenges the obscurity and bureaucracy of state welfare by exposing its contradictions...Advice to consumers on their entitlement, and advocacy to assist them to challenge unfair decisions has allowed welfare rights work to challenge the failure of state welfare schemes - in their own terms and under their own rules. It has demonstrated that consumers could take on the state welfare system, and win (Alcock, 1989: 35).

Alcock is effectively marrying the discourse of consumerism (markets) with that of entitlement (rights). The concept of welfare rights has been used most effectively in social security, where, as Alcock puts it 'obtuse legislation has prevented consumers from realising their entitlements to state welfare' (Alcock, 1989: 35). However, the concept could just as usefully be employed in areas of social care, in particular how disabled people gain access to social care services through community care assessments.

The dilemma for any disabled or older person attempting to assert their 'right' to social services is encapsulated by Biehal and colleagues:

> Many users of social services are excluded from full citizenship. Their right to treatment as equals may be limited by poverty, racism, assumptions about gender, age and disability. They often have no alternative but to depend on the decisions of welfare professionals, who control access to resources and exercise professional discretion about the use of these resources (Biehal et al, 1992: 109).

The problem has been highlighted by community care policy in the UK that explicitly leaves the discretion and the power in the use of resources in social care with the professionals - in this case, social services departments. Biehal and her colleagues see the solution to this problem as lying with social workers - placing the onus on them to prioritise the wishes and needs of services users over their own. However, within a welfare system where the professional gatekeepers exercise discretion, this type of self-regulation will not be sufficient to ensure that disabled people gain access to full citizenship through social rights.

Doyal and Harding (1992) posit an alternative solution. Access to social rights can be made meaningful, they argue, if disabled people can assert the right to procedural fairness against the gatekeepers who have the discretion over the use of resources. This approach does not ensure that services are available that will assist disabled people in their struggle for social citizenship, but they accept the limitations of this approach:

What community care suffers from above all is a political failure to make adequate provision on a fair and equitable basis. Procedural rights are no substitute for adequate policies, but they can address some of the injustices that currently beset community care. They can challenge inequalities, and bring a measure of dignity and respect to individuals. And by these means, they can help to focus public attention on the overriding failure of the political arrangements for community care. (Doyal and Harding, 1992: 73)

The key to procedural rights is, as in welfare rights, the method of gaining access to a service. Doyal and Harding point out that this hinges on whether or not potential services users have sufficient information to enable them to negotiate the system, and to know whether or not they are receiving fair treatment.

Citizenship, Negotiating Needs and Access to Services

This chapter has outlined the conceptual debate about citizenship that has informed social policy discourse over recent years. However, in this book I set out to adapt the concept of citizenship and use it to critically analyse the experiences of disabled people and their families who attempted to gain access to community care assessments. The citizenship framework will be developed further in subsequent chapters, but it is worth summarising it here to clarify the ensuing discussion.

Firstly, the Marshallian notion of civil and social rights, and the relationship between the two, will be developed further in chapter three and applied to the role of community care assessments as a means of gaining access to welfare goods. The way in which practitioners make decisions about who should access a community care assessment, and who should access services, will be placed in the context of the way in which the different rules and priorities for rationing access to scarce welfare goods are played out when competing claims for access to those goods are presented. The assessment process will be critically examined as one of the 'practices...which define a person as a competent member of society, and which as a consequence shape the flow of resources to persons and social groups' (Turner, 1993a: 2). In particular the way in which disabled people's civil and social rights are protected or threatened by the behaviour and decisions of practitioners acting as gatekeepers to scarce resources will be discussed in chapters four and five.

Secondly, the notion of a citizen being considered to be a 'competent member of society' will be used to critically examine the way in which competing definitions of need are presented and dealt with during the assessment process. Chapter six will discuss the way in which different participants in the process - potential 'users', 'carers' and the practitioner - had variable claims to being considered the 'most competent' person to assess the disabled person's needs for services and support. Thirdly, consideration will be given to the way in which the assessment process and outcome enables or prevents disabled people and their families from being competent 'members of society' - i.e. exercising choices and fulfilling what they conceived to be the duties of citizenship, a discourse sometimes referred to as social participation or exclusion.

3 Community Care for Disabled People in the 1990s

In this chapter I will discuss the various normative assumption behind the 1990s community care changes. I will examine the role that assessment was intended to play in community care policy, and discuss the normative core of community care policy. I will also expand on the concept of an assessment as a civil right, intended to unlock access to the social rights of community based services and support. I will show how the citizenship framework of civil and social rights originally envisaged by Marshall (1992) can be refined and adapted to analyse the status of disabled people needing services and support from their local authority.

The Community Care Changes

'Community care' is not a new policy. The closure of large scale 'workhouse' type units began with the inception of the National Health Service in 1948, although it did not become a major policy goal until the 1960s (Lewis and Glennerster, 1996). However, the impetus which led to the closure of long-stay hospitals and asylums in the 1960s and 1970s was rooted partly in the drive to reduce public expenditure and a reluctance to make large scale capital investments in institutional care and partly in a critical awareness of the quality of life experienced by people living in institutions (Townsend, 1962; Meacher, 1972). The impetus behind the 1990s changes has been argued to have a similar, but more refined focus, which included the drive to curb costs, the shift from public to private (and family) provision, and the facilitation of user empowerment.

Curbing Costs

During the 1970s, changes were made to the rules governing the allocation of social assistance benefits (Supplementary Benefit) to enable disabled people to claim discretionary supplements to help pay for the costs of residential care. Concerns at the level of discretionary power held by benefits officers led to pressure on central government to set up a defined system of rules and entitlements, which from November 1980 allowed full board and lodging costs in hostels and residential care to be claimed by lodgers (Lewis and Glennerster, 1996). Although probably intended to control expenditure, this move had the opposite effect. Between 1982 and 1992 social assistance expenditure on private residential and nursing home residents increased from £39m to £2,530m (Laing, 1993). The availability of social assistance funding also enabled other sectors of the welfare state (notably the NHS) to reduce its own provision for long-term care (Rummery and Glendinning, 1999).

Access to the additions to social assistance benefits to cover board and lodging were not based on any assessment of need, which explains the exponential rise in the numbers of recipients of these benefits. Lewis and Glennerster describe the effects of this policy:

> If you were a resident in [a residential home] and you had no more savings or capacity to pay, the social security system would meet your fees. If you did have savings and hoped to hand them onto your children why not do this at once, become officially poor and let the social security system pay the fees? If this had not occurred to you, a thoughtful owner of the old people's home was likely to put you in the picture (Lewis and Glennerster, 1996: 3).

In its review of the success of the shift of services from institutional to community-based care, the Audit Commission (1986) came to the conclusion that the perverse effect of social security policy was a major reason for the uneven development of community care. This was the explanation given for the lack of development of community-based alternatives to residential care (Bradshaw and Gibbs, 1988). However, this shift signified an important loss of rights for disabled people. Decisions made under social security legislation can be appealed against using the judicial system (usually through tribunals): there is no equivalent redress under the new community care arrangements (Glendinning, 1991). This is also in contrast to decisions made by social workers working with children under the 1989 Children's Act, which can be challenged within a judicial context.

Responsibility for both managing overall public spending on residential AND domiciliary services, and for assessing people's potential needs for those services, was given to social services departments with the full implementation of the 1990 Act in 1993. The introduction of assessment placed social services departments under an obligation to consider people's needs as well as their financial circumstances. This equated with an introduction of overt gatekeeping to social care services, via the assessment procedures put in place by each social services department.

In 1993, during the implementation of the new assessment arrangements, the Audit Commission issued a report which gave specific guidance to social services managers in drawing up the eligibility criteria for who should access assessments and services. Managers were advised that criteria should allow 'just enough people with needs to exactly use up their budget (or be prepared to adjust their budget)' (Audit Commission, 1993: para 15) to receive services. There is thus a clear onus on SSD mangers to control expenditure by controlling demand on resources, and the route set for them by central government to achieve that is by setting eligibility criteria for services very tightly.

However, whether or not people are eligible for services is likely to depend, largely, on whether they are viewed as needing them. In the previous chapter it was shown how the distinction between 'negative' civil rights and 'positive' social rights was based on the false premise that enforcing civil rights is cost neutral (Plant, 1990) Nevertheless, civil rights do differ in a significant way from social rights: civil rights are upholdable within a judicial context and subject to the rule of law, whereas social rights are rights to resources to meet needs. Because resources are not infinite, it follows that access to these resources must be gatekept. In this respect it cannot be said that disabled people have the civil right to access any services: it is not a right that can be upheld within a judicial context. The right to services to meet needs is therefore a social right, contingent on decisions made by whoever is responsible for carrying out gatekeeping.

Here the case of access to services, such as community care services in the UK, differs radically from the case of access to social security benefits in British social policy. The definition of need in the case of social security benefits, particularly income replacement benefits in the UK, is set centrally by national government. The criteria are applied at a local level by benefits officers working to nationally agreed guidelines. The rules (or eligibility criteria) are in many cases obscure, difficult to comprehend and act as a barrier that needs to be overcome by benefit applicants (Spicker, 1993) but they are upheld (and challenged) within a judicial context. Indeed, assisting benefits claimants to negotiate the eligibility criteria, and to appeal against discretionary decisions that do not appear to have been made within the rules is a key element of welfare rights work (Fimister, 1986; Alcock, 1989).

Defining need in community care is not so straightforward. Doyal and Gough point out that while most needs will be highly contested and socially and culturally contingent, it can still be meaningful to talk about universal needs. They envisage a hierachy of needs which flow from two universal needs: the need for physical survival, and the need for personal autonomy (Doyal and Gough, 1991). Within the social and cultural context of the UK in the 1990s, the rights accompanying these needs can be said to be the right to be free from personal harm and the right to minimally curtailed social participation in one's chosen form of life. Gaining access to services to meet these basic universal needs is crucial to the way disabled people gain access to citizenship: to how they become 'competent members of society' (Turner, 1993a: 2).

However, the concept of need within the policy and practice of community care does not accord with Doyal and Gough's concept of need. Indeed, the concept of need has proved to be one of the most problematic and contested concepts in community care. National policy guidance issued following the implementation of the 1990 Act was clear about the level of discretion that was assigned to local authorities in defining which needs they would agree to meet. It states that:

> Local authorities have a responsibility to meet needs within the resources available (Department of Health, 1990: 27).

Lewis and Glennerster point out the confusion engendered by the guidance issued to managers and practitioners prior to the full implementation of the 1990 Act (SSI/SSWG, 1991). Within that guidance, need is variously (and sometimes simultaneously) defined as 'complex', 'dynamic', 'multi faceted', defined both 'by the particular care agency or authority' while being a 'personal concept' (Lewis and Glennerster, 1996: 14). The most salient part of the managers' and practitioners' guidance apears to be the section which maintains that:

> Need is a dynamic concept, the definition of which will vary over time in accordance with: changes in national legislation; changes in local policy; *the availability of resources*; and patterns of local demand (SSI/SSWG, 1991: 12, emphasis added).

Thus in deciding which needs it will meet, and the eligibility criteria it will use, a local authority must align its definition of need with what needs it can afford to meet. In research carried out in five local authorities, Lewis and

Glennerster (1996) found that most of the eligibility criteria used by local authorities was tightly defined in relation to *risk*: people were only considered to be in need if they were at risk of harm to themselves or others. This is an indirect way of screening out as many applicants as possible, so that only those applicants whose needs the local authority can afford to meet fall within the eligibility criteria.

Recent legal rulings such as the Gloucestershire case (R v Gloucestershire CC and the Secretary of State for Health, ex parte Barry, 1997) have upheld the link between need and resources. The House of Lords decided that Gloucestershire County Council acted legally in withdrawing services it could not longer afford from a man who had previously been assessed as needing them. The 'universal principle' of curbing costs appears to be operating in place of the 'universal needs' of safety and personal autonomy.

Recalling the Audit Commission's exhortation to limit the number of people going through the system to roughly the number of people a local authority can afford to provide services for, it appears that there is an onus on both managers and front-line practitioners to balance their books in this way. Managers have to design and implement assessment systems designed to screen out as many people as possible, while ensuring that the system does not fail to pick up those people that are at risk. Front-line practitioners have to use their discretion to decide who should receive a full assessment of their needs, bearing in mind the cost restrictions on the level of services that can be offered.

This devolution of cost-curbing responsibility to managers and front-line practitioners is likely to have a significant effect on their practice. It is at odds with the professional ethics and standards of many social workers, who form the bulk of front-line practitioners (Cheetham, 1993; Braye and Preston-Shoot, 1995; Stevenson and Parsloe, 1993). Far from being a process of dialogue about uncovering needs, and establishing appropriate responses to them, the process of assessment is likely to be a process of balancing needs and resources (Challis, 1992). In this type of process there is little room for the reflexivity and anti-discriminatory practice that form the core values of social work practice (Sheppard, 1995). The onus is on front-line practitioners to apply managerial, budgetary control (Clarke and Newman, 1997), acting as street-level bureaucrats (Lipsky, 1980) rather than reflexive advocates.

Shifting Responsibility from the State to the Community

In examining the implementation of changes in policy it is helpful to establish the 'deep normative core' of the original policy. While Lewis and Glennerster's (1996) assertion that the 'deep normative core' of the community care changes was to curb expenditure carries some weight, the implementation of the changes was also a realization of another policy driver that had become apparent throughout the 1980s. This was the policy drive to shift the responsibility for *providing* care from the state to the community.

Until the beginning of the twentieth century, most of state provision of services for disabled people was institutional care. This carried with it the hallmark of stigma associated with state provision for paupers and those unable to work. However, even though they were living in institutional care, disabled people's families were still responsible for contributing to their upkeep. The 1930 Poor Law stated that:

> It should be the duty of the father, grandfather, mother, grandmother, husband or child, of a poor, old, blind, lame or impotent person, or other poor person, not able to work, if possessed of sufficient means, to relieve and maintain that person not able to work (quoted in Means and Smith, 1994: 19).

While not actually providing care or shelter, the community (in this case the disabled person's family) still had a responsibility for contributing financially towards his or her upkeep. Institutional care in the pre-Beveridge welfare state was actually a form of shared care between the community and the state.

In the Beveridge post-war model of the welfare state in the UK, institutional care was the main focus of provision for disabled and older people (Brown, 1972; Townsend, 1962). Means (1986) points out that one effect of this policy was that 'frail' disabled people were considered to be best cared for either in institutions, or by living with their families (i.e. daughters and daughters-in-law, if they were available). The concept of independent living in the community was not a feature of the early Beveridge welfare state.

Townsend's damning indictment of institutional (residential) care for disabled people (1962) was a key turning point in policy, although the recognition of the need to allow older disabled people to carry on living in their own homes as long as possible was a feature of policy aims much earlier (for example, see Ministry of Health, 1957). A key feature of this policy aim was a concern that the post-Beveridge welfare state had undermined family and community responsibility (Thompson, 1949), although concern for the decline in family care-giving was argued to be based on a myth (Lowther and Williamson, 1966). Townsend's detailed study of family care in London's East End in the 1950s (Townsend, 1963) showed that those older disabled people living in their own homes had extensive family resources, and that entering institutional care tended to be an option only for those people without those extensive family resources.

Means (1986) has detailed how state-provided domiciliary-based care was shown to be able to supplement care provided by families and reduce the need for institutional care. Similar conclusions were reached by Allen et al in their study of the views of older people in the community and in residential care (1992). The period between these two sets of conclusions was marked by the expansion in spending on residential care described above, so the two sets of conclusions need to be viewed from a relevant historical perspective. The case studies referred to by Means (1986) were written from the perspective of an era where little public expenditure went on domiciliary care or on supporting families to provide care for disabled people. Allen and her colleagues were writing from the perspective of the end of the 'golden age' of residential care where 'perverse incentives' prevented the development of domiciliary-based services. It should also be remembered that although the 'demographic time bomb' of an ageing population may be misleading (Hills, 1993) the numbers of both younger and older disabled people living in the community continue to rise, (for example, the Government's Actuary Department forecasts that the proportion of the UK's population over 65 will rise from 14% in 1951 to a forecasted 18% in 2001 and 24% on 2025) due in part to the improved health and living standards of the general population - arguably one of the successes of the post-war welfare state in the UK (Tinker, 1996). The cost of providing community and residential based care particularly for older disabled people looks set to continue to rise dramatically in the future (Richards, 1996).

The exponential growth in residential care in the 1980s looks, from the latter half of the 1990s, more like a historical blip in policy than an intended culmination of policy development. The community care changes do not look like the shifting of care from the state to the community, but the reassertion of the community as the dominant provider of care. While the 1989 White Paper Caring for People referred to 'care in the community' for disabled people, it might be more accurate to say that the policy was actually about 'care *by* the community'. In fact, the acknowledgement that a 'care in the community' policy actually meant the supporting of 'care by the community' had been made with regard to older people much earlier than Caring for People. The 1981 White Paper Growing Older asserted that:

> The primary sources of support and care for elderly people are informal and voluntary...It is the role of public authorities to sustain and, where necessary develop - but never to replace - such support and care. Care in the community means care by the community (DHSS, 1981).

What does care *by* the community mean? Who is the community? What are the implications of care by the community for the citizenship framework developed and used in this book? A closer analysis of the policy rhetoric and practice in community care reveals that the dominant discourse behind care by the community is in fact care provided by the family (Dalley, 1988) and that wider social networks play a much lesser part (Arber and Ginn, 1995). For the most part, this reflects research findings which have analysed the experience of caring for both care-givers and receivers and found that most help with the physical tending element of personal care (such as washing, dressing, medication, physical help and supervision) takes place within the context of the family (Townsend, 1963; Green, 1988).

However, it is too simplistic to delineate the close family as the sole source of support for many disabled and older people, as social networks provide other forms of support that are equally valued by disabled people even though only 7% of physical tending type care for older people comes from friends and neighbours (Green, 1988). The way in which community care policy is so overtly dependent on the bulk of the provision of care coming from the family does not necessarily resonate with the ways in which disabled people, and their families, conceive of themselves, their relationships and their obligations. Finch points out that:

Where social policies are designed to encourage a particular form of family responsibilities they are in fact seeking to create a particular moral order which may or may not accord with what people themselves actually feel is proper. (Finch, 1989: 8)

Thus, the normative assumption behind the community care changes (that the bulk of care *should* be provided by families) may well run into difficulties when it is applied to families who do not share that particular normative assumption, or whose definition of their obligations and 'proper' relationships differs from the state's.

Even the assertion that care by the community essentially means care by the family is not unproblematic. The 1980s saw an explosion of feminist analysis and research which attempted to account the gendered nature of the provision of care. These studies explored the experiences of women balancing childcare with caring for older relatives (Finch and Groves, 1983) carers who are daughters (Lewis and Meredith, 1988) and carers of disabled children (Glendinning, 1983). Feminist research explored the relationship between paid and unpaid caring (Graham, 1983) and the financial implications that caring has for women (Glendinning, 1992; Joshi, 1992; McLaughlin and Glendinning, 1994).

Viewed from the perspective of the citizenship framework used in this book, the issue of caring can be seen as the issue of the whether caring is construed as a way of an individual fulfilling their social duties and acting as a 'competent member of society' (Turner, 1993a). This is a question that cannot easily be separated from a feminist analysis of women's citizenship, as it is the way that caring has been conceived as women's work that has underpinned the development of the welfare state in the UK (Baldwin and Falkingham, 1994). One way in which the state has sought to support women's caring is through the payment of caring-specific benefits such as the Invalid Care Allowance (ICA) (although it took a struggle to make such benefits available to married women) which legitimises the carer-citizen by reimbursing them for their inability to be worker-citizen (McLaughlin and Glendinning, 1994). Feminist writers have welcomed the ICA as a citizenship benefit as it recognises the impact of caring on paid work while not policing the actual care given (Ungerson, 1992).

However, recognition of the loss of earnings is still not the same thing as reimbursing carers for the actual work of caring: it does not turn a carer-citizen into a worker-citizen (Lister, 1997). Feminist analysts have argued against paying carers for actual care tasks as this runs the risk of 'commodifying care' and relying on cheap, vulnerable women workers (Ungerson, 1993). However, as will be discussed below, allowing disabled people to employ their own carers using money that would otherwise have gone on local authority services has been a key demand of the disabled people's movement in the 1980s and 1990s, which resulted in the 1996 Community Care (Direct Payments) Act.

The strength of feminist work in this field has, until recently, obscured some of the other issues that are equally relevant to an analysis of community care and citizenship. Research carried out with spouse carers has highlighted that within these relationships many more men are providing care than had previously been acknowledged by feminist research: for example, in households where caring takes place, 59% of husbands and 71% of wives provide care (Arber and Ginn, 1995). Nevertheless, the nature of tasks still differs between the genders, with women more than twice as likely as men to be undertaking 'heavy duty' and intimate personal care (Arber and Ginn, op cit).

The feminist focus on what carers do has also obscured the way in which caring is often perceived by both the care-giver and recipient as a reciprocal relationship (Morris, 1991; 1996), particularly within spouse caring situations (Parker, 1993). It also obscured the way in which caring is viewed as a mark of citizenship. The experiences of disabled women who have been sterilized, and learning disabled women who have been either been prevented from becoming mothers, or whose care for their older parents has been ignored as their way of fulfilling their duties as a 'competent member of society', points to the value attached to being able to provide care when that cannot be taken for granted (Booth and Booth, 1994; Walmsley, 1993a). Disabled women have thus added another dimension to feminist concerns with caring and citizenship. It is not sufficient to view the caring/citizenship dilemma as being about how to recompense women for the loss of earnings and status that caring brings: citizenship may also be, for many women, a struggle for the right to care. This struggle has also been highlighted by Black feminist writers, who point out that the way in which the state seeks to problematise and control their caring has a significant impact on their citizenship status (hooks, 1982; Mama, 1992).

The normative core of the community care changes, shifting the provision of care from the state to the community, is therefore more complex that the policy rhetoric would seem to allow. Barnes (1997) points out that the Department of Health has quite deliberately left 'community' undefined in its policy and practice guidance, yet it is clear from the intended effects of the policy that the Department intended 'community' to be equivalent to 'family'. In doing so, they have adopted a normative core that is problematic and not necessarily shared by the families who are on the receiving end of the policy.

Faciliating User Empowerment

Although it would appear to be of secondary importance after the 'deep normative core' of curbing expenditure, the empowerment of service users does appear as a theme running through the rhetoric accompanying the community care changes. The 1989 White Paper Caring for People asserted that 'promoting choice and independence underlies all the government's proposals' (Department of Health, 1989; 4) and the guidance issued to social services managers and practitioners states that 'the rationale for this reorganisation is the empowerment of users and carers' (SSI/SSWG, 1991: 7).

The concept of empowerment, and its compatibility with the other, arguably overriding normative cores of community care policy is complex and contested (see for example Braye and Preston-Shoot, 1995; Stevenson and Parsloe, 1993; Barnes and Walker, 1996; Morris, 1997). The linguistic root of the word suggests that users will be given some power over the services they receive: this will involve removing some power from social services departments. However, the extent to which users have been granted power over the services they receive by the community care changes is limited. Some disabled writers have argued that social services departments have only engaged with the language of empowerment because they have been forced to do so following sustained pressure from service users (Oliver, 1990; Morris, 1991). Lobbying by groups of services users such as the British Council of Disabled People, Survivors Speak Out and People First, and direct challenges by individual service users have given users a 'voice' in the community care process. However, it is debatable how much power that voice has when pitted against the vested interests of local authorities.

Means and Smith (1994) argue that the push from service users towards greater empowerment is only likely to have a limited effect on the provision of services. It involves the challenging of professional stereotypes about disability (and old age), and replacing these with 'a deeper understanding of the problems faced by older people and people with disabilities' (Means and Smith, 1994: 75). This is difficult to achieve when groups of service users are diffuse, with different goals, agendas and epistemologies, and differentiated between organisations *of* and *for* disabled and older people. The lack of a politicised group of older service users, in contrast to some of the politicised groups of American older people (Pratt, 1993), also ameliorates the power that older disabled people have to challenge disempowering attitudes and behaviours on the part of practitioners.

In their defence, some writers have pointed out that anti-discriminatory practice, one of the 'core' values of social work, is one of the key drivers towards the empowerment of service users (Thompson, 1993). Braye and Preston-Shoot (1995) argue that practitioners should focus on empowering services users through ensuring equal access to services, and by adopting a radical social work perspective that maintains that the role of the practitioner should be to help service users overcome the discrimination they face in their lives. Sheppard (1995) views the role of the practitioner (within the care management process) as being one of partnership with the potential service user, thus empowering them. He asserts:

> The care management process becomes a partnership in which
> the practitioner and consumer bring different contributions: the
> practitioner their knowledge of available resources and ideas
> about their use; the consumer their capacity to decide, from a
> range of options, what they want...The practitioner's task is
> therefore twofold: helping the client define for themselves
> their need and helping them choose the best response to it.
> Their role is facilitating client choice (Sheppard, 1995: 101).

However, Sheppard's view of partnership does not appear to involve
the service user as an *equal* partner: they are not even considered to be
experts in defining their own needs, but to need a practitioner to help them
decide what their needs are. Cheetham agrees with Sheppard's view that the
role a practitioner plays in determining need is vital:

> Not all circumstances lend themselves to an articulate and systematic
> rehearsal of needs and most would agree that not all people, all of the time,
> are or should be the sole authority on their needs...Put crudely, do users' and
> carers' wishes for a service equal a need for it? An example, which will be
> highlighted by local authorities' new role as gatekeepers to residential care
> for those who require public funding, would be a request for a place in a
> residential home and the refusal of alternative intensive domestic support.
> (Cheetham, 1993: 164).

Cheetham has highlighted some of the key limitations of the aim of
empowering service users through the community care changes. Firstly, it is
practitioners working in social services departments who have the
information about the range of services available, and the criteria that
people have to fulfil to access the services. Myers and MacDonald (1996)
characterise five difficulties identified by practitioners in empowering
service users within this context: structural constraints; procedural
obstacles; cultural differences; practical difficulties and substantive
difficulties. They point out that when workers and users, or users and carers
disagree, many practitioners are faced with no other option than to assert
their professional dominance. Secondly, practitioners and their managers
are the budget holders, working within the explicit normative core,
discussed above, of curbing expenditure. The way in which social services
departments are the holders of all the money and information, and have the
responsibility for determining the definition of needs which it will meet has
been argued to be a key barrier in the empowerment of service users
(Stevenson and Parsloe, 1993).

The aim of user empowerment is also in conflict with the second
normative core of the community care changes, discussed above, of shifting

the provision of care from the state to the community. The 1989 White Paper Caring for People was explicit in the way that it set out one of the key aims of the community care reforms as being the support of carers. Yet it glossed over how this aim could be reconciled with the empowerment of service users. Cheetham points out the dilemma that she felt would face practitioners implementing the community care reforms:

The concept of partnership will be tested in the community care triangle of carer, user and social worker. In their assessments of need, and particularly in any equation between these and resource plans or requests, social workers will have painful choices to make in the priority they think should be accorded to carers' needs when these may conflict with the needs, or at least the wishes, of a person being cared for. (Cheetham, 1993: 165)

Of course, an overriding concern with how to reconcile the conflicting needs of users and carers overlooks the fact that many users and carers do not feel that their needs and identities fall into this dichotomy. As discussed above, many people (particularly spouses) experience providing and receiving care as a reciprocal relationship (Arber and Ginn, 1995) and many disabled people, who would be seen as service users, view themselves as having caring responsibilities (Morris, 1991). However, it has been shown that in situations where there may be conflict over needs, the person with the better communication skills will tend to dominate the process of negotiation (Wertheimer, 1993) which may have consequences for the empowerment of the person less able to communicate their wishes. From a citizenship perspective, the person who practitioners perceive as the most 'competent member of society' may find that they have to compete with people perceived as less 'competent' to define and articulate their needs. Services designed to support one party in fulfilling their social duties and acting as a social being may mitigate against the other party's social participation. The issue of who is considered competent to assess needs, and therefore who is treated as a 'citizen' within the assessment process is explored more fully in chapters four (from the perspective of practitioners) and six (from the perspective of disabled people and their families).

Thirdly, even using the Department of Health's narrow conceptualisation of empowerment as being about choice for users, there are key obstacles to the goal of user empowerment within the community care reforms. The reforms introduced market mechanisms into social care as a means of offering service users the choice between alternative services and the opportunity to affect the quality of services through being able to exit from poor quality providers (Hoyes et al, 1993). However, commentators have pointed out that the social care market (despite the fact that it operates as a fully mixed market; i.e. services are purchased from a mix of statutory and independent providers) operates at most as a quasi-market (LeGrand and Bartlett, 1993). The consumer who has the choice of which provider to purchase from, and who has the option of exit from contracts to ensure quality, is not the service user but the social services department, on their behalf.

This means that service users cannot be said to be empowered by the option of exercising choice of providers, or being able to exit and change providers. The only real choice they have is to refuse to accept the services that are offered and attempt to make their own arrangments, which, given the lack of information most service users can easily obtain about alternative providers, and the cost implications of privately arranging care is likely to only be a realistic option for a small proportion of users (Baldock and Ungerson, 1993; Bosanquet and Propper, 1991; Mackintosh et al, 1990). However, as will be argued in chapter six, giving disabled people money instead of services does enable them to exercise a limited about of consumerist power.

Nevertheless, many service users would find the idea of themselves as consumers a mockery of the debilitating effects they consider being service users has had upon their lives and would characterise themselves as 'survivors' of services rather than 'consumers' of them (Barnes et al, 1990). At its best, it is the social services manager who is empowered by the introduction of market mechanisms into social care, rather than the service user: but the manager is not the intended beneficiary of the services, nor were the reforms intended to empower her. Even where the service user can exercise some control over the way in which they receive services, as in the case of direct payments, it is still the practitioner who decide on the level of need and thus level of payment. Barnes (1997) argues that the difficulties with the market approach to social care make the term 'consumer' misleading: not only are social care markets 'quasi-markets' but service users are 'quasi-consumers'. However, it is arguable whether service users are consumers at all.

In implementing the reforms many local authorities recognised the limitations of the market approach in empowering service users. They sought to position themselves as 'market enablers', by both stimulating the mixed market and seeking to enable the personal development of both individual service users and communities through allowing citizens a voice in a democratic process (Wistow and Barnes, 1995). Thus, local authorities seek to empower service users through giving them a voice in the consultation process around community care plans (Bewley and Glendinning, 1994) and through giving them a voice in the assessment and care management process (Braye and Preston-Shoot, 1995; Stevenson and

Parsloe, 1993). Barnes (1999) has argued that the 'democratic' approach to empowerment is a more powerful means of empowering service users than a market approach. However, Bewley and Glendinning, in their study of consultation with service users around community care plans, noted that difficulties such as the 'representativeness' of the people consulted (particularly the low rates of consultation with older disabled people or groups of older people, and similarly with people with sensory impairments) and issues raised by disabled people and their organisations concerning the effectiveness and usefulness of their involvement mean that the democratic approach to empowerment is not unproblematic (Bewley and Glendinning, 1994).

Finally, Morris (1997) questions whether or not the key concepts of the reforms, care and empowerment, are actually mutually exclusive. She asserts that:

> Empowerment means choice and control; it means that someone has the power to exert choice and therefore maximise control in their lives (always recognising that there are limits to how much control any of us have over what happens in our lives). Care - in the second half of the twentieth century - has come to mean not caring about someone but caring for in the sense of taking responsibility for. People who are said to need caring for are assumed to be unable to exert choice and control. One cannot, therefore, have care and empowerment, for it is the ideology and the practice of caring which has led to the perception of disabled people as powerless (Morris, 1997:54).

Thus the explicit and implicit normative cores of community care policy, curbing costs and shifting the provision of care to the community, are in conflict with the aim of empowering disabled and older people. Putting control of resources into professionals' rather than disabled and older people's hands, and explicitly supporting family care, are perpetuating what Brisenden refers to as 'the most exploitative' relationship-ruining form of care provision (Brisenden, 1989), which Morris maintains directly contravenes any notion of empowerment or civil rights.

If we examine Morris' concepts of 'choice and control' from a citizenship perspective, then it is clear from her analysis that the discourse of caring assumes that a disabled person receiving care is unable to discharge their citizenship duties and act as a 'competent member of society'. Being able to exercise choice and control can be linked to Doyal and Gough's (1991) assertion that one of the basic rights associated with citizenship is the right to minimally curtailed participation in one's chosen form of life - otherwise referred to as 'social participation'. By deliberately placing the locus of the exercising of choice and control in the hands of the practitioner rather the service user, the community care reforms have protected the status of the practitioner as citizen over the status of the user as citizen. The implications of this will be explored further in chapters four and six which will discuss the issue of how the assessment process treats the various participants as 'competent' or not to decide need and assert claims to services, and in how the results of that process affect the abilities of disabled people and their families to exercise choice and control in the way they fulfil their citizenship duties and participate in society.

Assessment and Citizenship

In the final section of this chapter, the role of assessment in the community care reforms, and its relationship to the citizenship framework used in this book will be discussed. This is a useful point to revisit and develop some of the key concepts and themes touched on in chapter two, particularly Marshall's concept, developed by Plant (1990, 1992) and Lister (1995, 1997) among others, of the difference between civil and social rights and the way in which that is applied to the assessment process.

The Civil Right to an Assessment Versus the Social Right to Services

Marshall (1992) argued that political, civil and social rights developed sequentially and characterise the evolution of the relationship between the citizen and the state. Political rights give the individual leverage over the state, by allowing her to vote for or against the government. Civil rights have resulted from the growth in the rule of law and legal rights, and are concerned with granting the individual protection both from other individuals and from the excesses of state power. According to Marshall's framework, social rights confer upon individuals equality of status through the provision of resources to meet need. He was clear that this provision was never intended to lead to equality of outcomes: the fact that the state undertook to meet basic needs was intended to make inequality of outcomes less divisive and important.

One particular element of Marshall's framework is useful in accounting for the role of assessment and gatekeeping in the community care reforms. His account of the difference between civil and social rights, and thus civil and social citizenship, highlights an important dimension of the relationship between assessment and disabled people's citizenship. Civil rights are bound by the rule of law: that is, they apply equally to the representatives of the state and to individuals, and they must be clearly challanged or upheld within a judicial context. Social rights, on the other hand, are rights to resources to meet needs.

Applying the Marshallian framework to assessment within community care, the right to an assessment is actually a civil right for many disabled people. It is enshrined in and protected by the judicial system of the UK. Under s4 of the 1986 Disabled Persons (Services, Consultation and Representation) Act, disabled people have the right to access an assessment of their needs. This right applies if the applicant falls into the definition of 'disabled person' laid down in the 1948 National Assistance Act, i.e.: people aged eighteen or over who are blind, deaf or dumb, or who suffer from mental disorder of any description and other persons aged eighteen or over who are substantially and permanently handicapped by illness, injury or congenital deformity or such other disabilities as may be prescribed by the minister.

Local authorities have been advised to interpret 'substantially' as widely as possible (Department of Health, 1993; Mandelstam and Schwer, 1995). There is no upper age limit to a disabled person's right to access an assessment, a point which will become significant in chapter four. The right granted under the 1986 Act has also not been superseded by the 1990 NHS and Community Care Act: s47 of the 1990 Act actually placed additional duties on social services departments to assess not only disabled people but anyone who appeared to be in need of the services that they provide. This civil right does have cost implications: social services departments clearly have a duty to employ people to carry out assessments. However, the fact that it has cost implications does not, as has been argued in chapter two, preclude it from being a civil, rather than a social right.

There is no civil right to any particular social care service. In fact, there is also no civil right to any particular health care service or intervention: a person's ability to access services is contingent on the professional judgement of a clinician. Similarly, in social care, a person's right to access services to meet their needs is contingent on the professional judgement of a social services assessor. Salter (1994) has attempted to argue that the community care reforms signalled a shift from universal (NHS) rights to health care to contingent rights to social care. However, the role of clinical discretion in professional gatekeeping to health care services is not so very different from the role of practitioner discretion in professional gatekeeping to social care services under the post-community care reforms system of assessment (Rummery and Glendinning, 1999). Both are gatekeeping access to resources to meet the needs of claimants.

Gatekeeping and Rationing in Social Care

The way that professional discretion is used to gatekeep access to services within the British welfare state is in contrast to the way in which professional discretion is minimised in accessing many income-replacement and other cash benefits in the UK. Benefit levels are for the most part set nationally, and the criteria for accessing benefits (for both insurance and means-tested benefits) is determined and applied nationally. Indeed, appeals against decisions made by Department of Social Security benefits officers applying the criteria to individual applicant cases are made in a judicial context, through the use of tribunals. Applying the Marshallian framework of rights developed above, benefits can thus be said to be civil rights, even though they are rights to resources. It is for this reason that most of the current work around citizenship within the discipline of social policy is being applied to anti-poverty work (Mead, 1997; Lister, 1997). Welfare rights work has thus been able to uphold and protect citizen's rights by challenging social security decisions using legal principles of judicial review (Alcock, 1989; Fimister, 1986).

The case of accessing services, rather than benefits, to meet needs is more ambiguous. Decisions are more obviously highly contingent on the discretion of professionals. The criteria for accessing community care services are not set nationally: local authority social services departments were given explicit discretion in setting the criteria within their own budgetary limitations. There is, as discussed earlier in this chapter, a clear onus on social services managers to manage demand for services by setting criteria very tightly. There is also a clear onus on front-line practitioners to manage demand through the assessment process: their role, post 1993, is clearly about rationing access to services (Lewis and Glennerster, 1996; Ellis, 1995).

Rationing is an emotive, unpopular term (Klein et al, 1996). It conjures up images of wartime privations and, more recently, of expensive health care being denied to sick children. Nevertheless, while the word does not appear in any of the community care legislation or accompanying guidance, the earlier section on curbing costs argued that rationing access to finite resources was the 'deep normative core' of the community care reforms. The assessment process is an overt rationing tool.

This is not, in itself, problematic for disabled people's citizenship. Marshall accepted that social rights were rights to resources, and were necessarily contingent upon professional gatekeeping. However, the assessment process can be conceptualized as the arena in which applicants and professional gatekeepers negotiate access to services to meet needs: the arena for the negotiation of social rights. Therefore, the way in which these social rights are negotiated is a crucial issue for the citizenship status of disabled people. Chapters four and six will explore this issue in more depth.

There is perhaps an even more crucial issue: how disabled people gain access to the negotiating arena in the first place. Social rights are very difficult to protect if applicants face barriers in actually getting to the stage of presenting their needs to professional gatekeepers. A vital part of the exploration of disabled people's citizenship status in community care is therefore examining whether or not their civil right to the assessment itself is upheld by the process. Marshall's view of social rights evolving directly out of civil rights may have resonance in community care: disabled people's social rights to services to meet their needs are obviously going to depend on their civil right to an assessment being protected. The type of barriers which social services departments use to gatekeep access to assessments, and the implications those barriers have for disabled people's civil rights, are explored in the next chapter.

4 Managing Demand at the Frontline: Managerial, Bureaucratic and Professional Gatekeeping

The previous two chapters showed how the Marshallian notion of civil and social rights can be applied to community care assessments and services - the former being a civil right and the latter a social right. This chapter will now address the question of how frontline practitioners make decisions about who gets access to community care assessments and services - how does the way in which they manage demand for assessments and services impact upon the civil and social rights of disabled people and their families? And how do practitioners balance the sometimes competing claims to be the most competent person to assess a disabled person's needs: whose views are given the greatest legitimacy, and why? The chapter will begin by describing the structure and function of the six teams that took part in the study. It will then briefly describe the formal criteria and procedures laid down by managers across each local authority.

However, as will become clear, the behaviour and decision-making processes employed by front-line practitioners in deciding who should access an assessment, and who then should access services, was only slightly influenced by the formal criteria and procedures set down in their staff manuals. Of far greater significance was the type of team (delineated by both the user group served by the team, and the team's culture and values) in which practitioners worked. For this reason, the bulk of this chapter is based on observations of actual assessment practice (see Davis et al, 1997 for details of the research methods).

The Structure of Assessment Services in the Two Local Authorities

Local authority A was a metropolitan borough council with a predominantly urban population of 302,500. 9.7% of their residents were from ethnic minority communities. Assessment services were provided by Assessment and Care Management Teams which had a specialist focus (older people, younger disabled people, people with sensory impairments) which complemented other specialist teams (mental health and learning disabilities). The team for older people was split into four geographical areas of the city: the other assessment teams covered the whole city. The only exception to this was the hospital social work team, who were based in the city's one large hospital. They provided assessment (plus six weeks care management) services to all patients in the hospital who were not currently receiving active assessment or care management services from one of the community based teams. Table 4.1 shows the client group of the three teams in local authority A who took part in the study:

Table 4.1   Team client groups in local authority A

Team	Client group
The Hospital Team of	Patients in hospital in local authority A who were about to be discharged, and were not 'open' to any the community teams.
The Younger Person's Team	Disabled people between the ages of 18 and 65 living in local authority A and not: • mentally ill, • learning disabled or • sensory impaired
The Older Person's Team	Disabled people over the age of 65 living in the northern section of local authority A and not: • mentally ill • learning disabled or • sensory impaired

Local authority B was a large county council with a mixture of urban and rural population. Its population was 498,563, of which 3.4% came from ethnic minority communities. Apart from specialist mental health and learning disabilities teams, assessment services were provided by area based generic social work teams, supplemented by two sensory impairment teams that covered the whole county. The observations in this local authority did not cover any of the hospital social work teams. Table 4.2 shows the client group of the three teams in local authority B that took part in the study:

Table 4.2   Team client groups in local authority B

Team	Client group
The Generic Team	Disabled people over the age of 18 living in one of five sections of county B who were not: • mentally ill • learning disabled or • sensory impaired
The Deaf Team	Deaf children and adults living in local authority B.
The Blind Team sighted	People being registered as blind and partially in local authority B - and unregistered or already registered blind and partially sighted people

Figure 4.1   Flow of cases for assessment and care management in local authority A

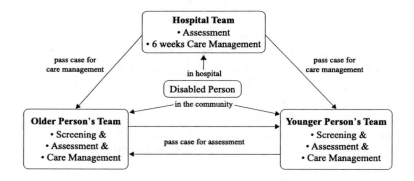

The flow of cases from initial enquiry until the point of assessment across teams in each of the local authorities is shown in figures 4.1 and 4.2.

Figure 4.2   Flow of cases for assessment and care management in local authority B

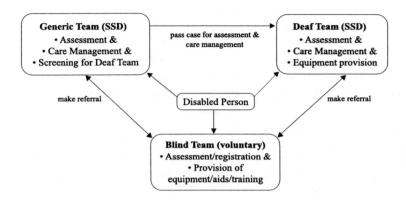

Local authority A's organisation did not fit easily within any one model of assessment organisation proposed by central government. In guidance issued to social services managers prior to the implementation of the 1990 Act (SSI/SSWG, 1991) nine organisational models were described. Briefly, these were:

(1) A two tier model separating information and advice from actual assessments;
(2) A differentiated model where reception staff sometimes provide information, and users are sometimes allocated for a full assessment according to need;
(3) A specialist assessment model, whereby practitioners provide assessments either within (a) a generic team (b) a specialist user/client focused team (c) a specialist user/client focused team with provider input or (d) a specialist resource centre;
(4) Sub-contracting assessment to a specialist agency;
(5) Splitting assessment from care planning;
(6) Splitting assessment from purchasing;
(7) Combining assessment with purchasing;
(8) Combining assessment with service provision; and
(9) Integrating assessment with (a) other core tasks of care management or (b) other core tasks for people with complex needs, delegating simpler core tasks to other staff (SSI/SSWG, 1991: 51-54).

These models do not seem to be intended to be either overly

prescriptive or exclusive. If local authority A's managerial structure is compared to the SSI/SSWG models it becomes clear that no one model was adopted authority-wide: rather, each team bore some similarities to one or more of the models. Authority-wide, the use of the Older Person's Teams to screen referrals and pass cases for assessment onto specialist teams suggests they are operating something like a combination of models (2), (3) (a) and (7). However, the specialist teams in local authority A, such as the Younger Person's Team, seemed to be operating in a way more like a combination of models (2) and (3) (d) and (7). On the other hand, the Hospital Team seemed to act like model (7), keeping all assessment and care management tasks within the team, with some elements of model (9) in that some members of the team only dealt with people with complex needs needing a comprehensive assessment, whereas others carried out all screening, assessment and care management tasks for those with lower level needs.

Similarly, the organisation of local authority B as a whole did not reflect any one SSI/SSWG model, and it is easier to compare the managerial structure to the SSI/SSWG models on a team by team basis. The Generic Team operated a like model (2) in the way it screened cases for the specialist teams, and a combination of model (7) in the assessments it carried out itself, and model (8) in the way it passed some low-level assessments to home care managers (see section on generic teams below for a further explanation of this). The Deaf Team operated very like model (3) (d), with some elements of model (7) in the way that assessors also acted as care managers. The Blind Team was the only team that worked in a way approaching model (4), because of the way assessment functions had been subcontracted to them as a voluntary agency by the local authority B's social services department. The rehabilitation officers in the Blind Team also worked like model (8) in the way they combined the provision of services, equipment and training with assessment (see section on specialist teams below).

Managerial Gatekeeping

All the teams operated with managerially defined criteria which defined who should get access to an assessment. Because these criteria were set by managers, and meant to be applied universally by all practitioners regardless of which team they were working, within this book they have been designated as 'managerial gatekeeping', reflecting the 'new managerialist' pressures on local authority social services managers (Clarke and Newman, 1997). It places social services managers under pressure to take responsibility for reducing public expenditure while still theoretically applying 'needs-based' criteria for accessing assessments and services (Blackman, 1999). The only exception to the universality of these criteria was the way that the Blind Team operated, because they were a voluntary organisation they did not use local authority B's eligbility criteria. In fact, this made no difference to their practice, as they carried out assessments on everyone that was referred to them (see below under specialist teams section for an explanation of this).

The eligibility criteria were published in both staff manuals and, in an abridged or simplified form, in leaflets that were available to the public in the reception areas of the team offices. They were set by senior managers, not the team managers, and renewed or altered annually in line with budgetary pressures. At the time of the research the staff manual in local authority B was considered out of date as it had not been updated in the light of a recent reorganisation of social work teams and providers. Consequently, the staff manual was referred to with much greater frequency by practitioners in local authority A. Nevertheless, practitioners in local authority B did use their staff manual to check the eligibility criteria on occasion, so their eligibility criteria are reproduced below.

As discussed earlier, these eligibility criteria are, following government guidance (SSI/SSWG, 1991) specifically designed to ensure that teams are not faced with unmanageable demand for services. By controlling the numbers of people who gain access to an assessment, managers are controlling demand for services, as both staff manuals were clear that services could only be provided without an assessment in the most exceptional circumstances (usually because a person was considered to be at risk and it was considered dangerous to wait for an assessment).

Local authority A's eligbility criteria for accessing a community care assessment is reproduced in table 4.3.

Table 4.3   Eligibility criteria in local authority A

Who is eligible for an assessment?	People who are 'vulnerable' or are asking for an assessment under the 1986 Disabled Person's Act
When is this decided?	During 'screening' undertaken by a duty social worker or welfare assistant
Are there different levels of assessment?	Yes, 3 levels of assessment according to the level of risk and whether or not applicants have 'complex' needs

One of the most significant factors about local authority A's eligibility criteria is that they explicitly refer to a disabled person's right, under the 1986 Disabled Persons (Services, Consultation and Representation) Act, to request an assessment of their needs. The acknowledgement of this right in the formal staff procedures manual meant that all practitioners were at least nominally aware of disabled people's right to an assessment. The reason that this is significant will become clear later in this chapter.

Local authority B's eligibility criteria (both social services', and the Blind Team's) are reproduced in table 4.4 below:

Table 4.4   Eligibility criteria in local authority B

	Local authority B SSD	**Blind Team**
Who is eligible for an assessment?	People at immediate or imminent risk of harm, who have insufficient informal care - people at a 'lower' risk will only be assessed once everyone at the 'higher' level of risk has received services	People who are blind or partially sighted
When is this decided?	During the 'initial' assessment undertaken by the duty social worker	By the receptionist on the initial enquiry
Are there different levels of assessment?	Yes, according to how many levels of the computerised record system need to be filled in. After the 'initial' assessment, a 'further' assessment is carried out if the person ends up receiving services, and a 'full' assessment if some liaison with other agencies is necessary, or a complicated 'package' of services is needed.	No

There are two notable differences between the social services eligibility criteria used by local authority B as compared to local authority A. Firstly, there was no explicit mention of a disabled person's right to access an assessment under the 1986 Disabled Persons (Services, Consultation and Representation) Act: awareness of this right was therefore down to the training and knowledge of individual practitioners. Secondly, local authority B explicitly designated the presence of what was considered by practitioners to be a 'sufficient' level of informal care as a reason for finding applicants for community care assessments to be at a 'lower' risk level. As will become clear from the evidence presented later in this chapter, practitioners would often judge whether an applicant for an assessment had 'sufficient' informal care on the basis of very little information, and their definition of 'sufficient' would often not coincide with the views of a disabled applicant. People with 'carers' were therefore prevented from accessing an assessment until all the people without 'carers' had been assessed: but the people designated as 'carers' would not necessarily be considered carers by either themselves or the disabled people applying for assessments.

During the course of the study, it became obvious that there was no clear delineated point at which decisions about whether or not a person should access an assessment ended and the assessment itself began. Practitioners in all the teams verified during feedback sessions that this was the case: because it was practitioners, rather than reception staff, who were for the most part screening initial enquiries and requests for assessments, the information gathering part of the assessment began at the point of enquiry.

However, practitioners in all the teams operated differentiated levels or tiers of assessment. What was clear from the evidence was that the managerial gatekeeping mechanisms of official eligibility criteria bore very little relationship to the day to day practice of practitioners. Decisions made by practitioners about a person's level of need, and thus the level of assessment needed, bore more similarity to decisions made by practitioners in similar type teams in the other local authority, rather than practitioners in other teams within the same local authority. Practitioners in all the teams were acting like street-level bureaucrats (Lipsky, 1980) in the way they made decisions about whether or not an application warranted a further assessment or services, and the way that they used their decision making about people's needs to manage demand for services. For this reason, the following section describes the way that teams across the two local authorities fell into three team types, and the sections discussing the methods used by practitioners to manage demand for services by gatekeeping access to assessments is entitled 'bureaucratic gatekeeping'.

Classification of Team Types

This section will group together the six teams in the study, and briefly describe the characteristics common to each team type. This section is intended as an introduction designed to make sense of the following section on 'bureaucratic gatekeeping' rather than an in-depth examination of the organisation and values of each team type.

Hospital

When the observations of assessment practice in the Hospital Team was compared to the other five teams, it became clear that practitioners in the Hospital Team were responding to pressures that were unique to their team. Consequently, decisions about what level of assessment patients should access, and which services they should receive, were made according to values and ways of working which were direct responses to those pressures.

Practitioners and managers in the Hospital Team were under an obligation to carry out assessments on every patient in hospital who was referred to them, because these patients were waiting to be discharged into the community. Under the terms of the Special Transitional Grant, health authorities and social services departments had to have agreed hospital discharge procedures for those patients considered to need social care services by December 1992. The discharge procedures agreed between local authority A and the relevant health authority meant that all patients referred to the team had to be visited by a duty social worker to carry out an initial assessment of need, to establish what level of assessment and services were needed for the patient to be discharged.

Consequently, every patient referred to the team accessed an assessment, although this assessment was sometimes very brief. Practitioners in this team did not have an individual budget for each service user, but used the team budgets of the relevant community based team in local authority A. They needed the team leader's permission to set up services, but this was never refused during the course of the study. Consequently, practitioners in this team were not under the same kind of direct pressure to ration access to resources and services as practitioners in other teams, just as Social Fund officers without budgetary constraints did not allow rationing to dominate their decision making in the way they did when they were under direct budgetary constraint (Huby and Dix, 1992).

Specialist

The Younger Person's Team, the Deaf Team and the Blind Team all fell within the specialist team type. They had a specialist client group focus of, respectively, disabled people under 65, deaf people and blind and partially sighted people. Perhaps partly because nearly all the applicants to these teams would fit within the legal definition of disabled and thus have the right to ask for an assessment of their needs, everyone approaching these teams accessed a community care assessment.

The Blind Team's client group were comprised mainly of people who were either in the process of being registered blind or partially sighted, or had already been registered. The registration process is an official process, set in motion by a hospital consultant, which changed a person's status in various ways: it makes them eligible for certain tax credits, benefits and invalidates their driving licence. It is not compulsory (although once the consultant has filled in the relevant certificate, people will find their car insurance is invalidated and so, legally, they cannot drive anyway) but it is necessary in order to gain access to the tax credits and other benefits. The Blind Team registered approximately 2,300 people as blind, and 380 people as partially sighted in local authority B each year. Because the process is a formal, statutory process, everyone who is eligible for registration accesses a full assessment. The Blind Team extended this service to people referred to the team who were not being registered blind or partially sighted.

There were therefore no appreciable barriers to accessing an assessment in either the hospital or specialist teams, other than a person's age or impairment. In addition, the specialist teams all made explicit reference in procedures manuals, posters on walls and literature available to service users, to the social model of disability (Oliver, 1990; Barnes, 1991). This is a sociological model of disability that has grown from the independent living and disability movements in the USA and the UK (UPIAS, 1976). It maintains that people with impairments or chronic illnesses are disabled by the physical, environmental and attitudinal barriers that they face in society: it places the locus of the problem in society, rather than in disabled people's impairments or illnesses. Although this model has been critiqued by both mainstream sociologists (Williams, 1991) and from within the disability movement for failing to take into account issues of gender (Morris, 1992) and race (Stuart, 1993), it has proved to be an enduringly popular model with the disability movement. The specialist teams also all employed disabled practitioners, which was not the case in either the hospital or generic/older person's teams.

Practitioners in these teams were not working with budget limits for each service user, but within team budget limits. It was therefore their managers' responsibility, rather than their own, to ensure that packages of care for service users did not go over budget limits. Individual practitioners were aware of certain budgetary restraints, such as the 'ceiling' of the weekly cost of residential care, and another 'ceiling' of how much per week would be available under the Independent Living Fund, and these did not appear in practice to be negotiable (for example the fieldwork notes reveal no instances where a practitioner negotiated with a manager to spend more than the 'ceiling' allowed for domiciliary care: all such cases observed seemed to be automatically referred for residential care). However, practitioners in these teams tended, more than the other teams, to be able to access different funding and service sources for service users, such as the Independent Living Fund, local charitable networks or (particularly in the case of the Blind Team) stocks of equipment and access to training. The section on professional gatekeeping will explore the relationship between these alternative funding and service sources on the practitioners' decisions about disabled people's needs.

Generic/Older

The situation in the Older Person's Team and the Generic team was very different from that in the hospital and specialist teams. These teams had potentially the largest client base: the Older Person's team screened most of the initial enquiries for the specialist teams and carried out assessments for all older people and younger people with HIV and AIDS in the locality; and the Generic Team screened many initial enquiries for the specialist teams and carried out assessments for all disabled people over 18 living in the locality.

Teams of this type did not allow all applicants to access a community care assessment. Instead, the onus was placed on front-line practitioners to manage the demand for services by gatekeeping access to assessments. They did this by using the discretion allowed to them by the system to employ a variety of bureaucractic gatekeeping mechanisms (Lipsky, 1980) which are discussed below. In employing these mechanisms, front-line practitioners are behaving in way that has become an established phenomenon in social policy: behaving as rationers. This has been observed in many areas of public provision, whether it be Social Fund officers changing their behaviour, refusal rates and definitions of needs when placed under budgetary constraints (Huby and Dix, 1992) or housing officers failing to make known the criteria for allocating housing in their borough, or making the criteria difficult to fulfill and using waiting lists to deter people (Institute of Housing, 1990). Although rationing is an emotive term (and one rejected by the front-line practitioners in this study as a explanation of their behaviour) Klein et al (1996) assert that the discretionary power held by front-line practitioners to employ these mechanisms is a way of managing demand and therefore rationing access to services and resources.

Practitioners in the Generic Team were using a computerised information system which limited how much they were allowed to spend on services for each service user: unlike the hospital and specialist teams, and the Older Person's Team, where decisions about whether the cost of service packages for users could be afforded were made by team managers rather than individual practitioners. This appeared to place practitioners in the Generic Team under additional pressure to gatekeep access to resources, which might explain their more extensive use of bureaucratic gatekeeping mechanisms than the other teams.

Controlling Access to Assessments through Bureaucratic Gatekeeping

As discussed above, only the generic/older person's teams used gatekeeping access to assessments as a mechanism for managing demand for services and resources. If the assessment is the arena in which needs and access to resources to meet those needs (i.e. people's social rights) are negotiated, then failing to access an assessment (people's civil right) will obviously have worrying consequences for disabled people. In contrast, the hospital and specialist teams allowed every applicant to access an assessment from a practitioner in the team, and so used other mechanisms (discussed in the section on professional gatekeeping) during the assessment itself to manage the demand for services and resources. This section will therefore concentrate in the mechanisms used by managers and front-line practitioners in the generic/older person's teams to manage the demand for assessments.

The Right to an Assessment?

Local authority B (and therefore the Generic Team) did not make any explicit reference to disabled people's right to access a community care assessment under the 1986 Act in their procedures manual. Practitioners in that team did not appear to be aware of that right in the same way as practitioners in other teams, particularly in local authority A, which did make explicit reference to that right in their procedures manual. As has been pointed out by other commentators (Doyle and Harding, 1992; Biehal et al, 1992) the concept of a 'right' to any welfare service becomes meaningless when front-line practitioners are not aware of the duties they are placed under according to that right.

However, practitioners in the Deaf Team were working with the same procedures as the Generic Team, and they did behave as though people approaching them with enquiries had the right to access a community care assessment. Similarly, practitioners in the Older Person's Team in local authority A, whose procedures manual did explicitly refer to disabled people's right to access a community care assessment, behaved as though the people approaching them with enquiries did not have that right. One possible explanation for this is the fact that people approaching the Older Person's Team were mostly over 65, and thus deemed to be 'older' rather than 'disabled'. The right to an assessment under the 1986 Disabled Persons (Services, Consultation and Representation) Act has no upper age limit. Policy guidance on the NHSCCA explicitly reasserts disabled people's rights to an assessment under the 1986 Act, and places local authorities under an obligation to inform enquirers to whom this Act applies of their rights (Department of Health, 1990: 28 para 3.30).

However, it also difficult to establish from the evidence how much of the hospital team's insistence on assessing everyone who was referred to them was down to disabled people's right to access an assessment (which they were aware of as it featured in their procedures manual), and how much was down to their obligations to the health authority under the continuing care agreement. As most of the hospital team's client groups were over 65, I would suggest that it was the latter rather than the former which dictated that everyone received an assessment.

Bureaucratic Barriers to an Assessment

Practitioners in the generic/older person's teams used a variety of mechanisms to control the demand for assessments. The disabled people and carers interviewed for this study who accessed an assessment from the Generic Team experienced these mechanisms as barriers, sometimes quite significant and difficult to overcome, to accessing an assessment, and therefore to accessing services to meet their needs (see chapter six).

Klein et al (1996) have developed Parker's (1975) typology of rationing to describe seven types of rationing mechanisms to control the demand for public services. These are: rationing by denial, where would-be beneficiaries are turned away on the grounds that their needs are not genuine or urgent enough; rationing by selection, where services are concentrated on those most likely to benefit; rationing by deflection, where would-be beneficiaries are steered towards another agency or provider of services; rationing by deterrence, where access to the system is made difficult for applicants; rationing by delay, for example by using a waiting list; rationing by dilution, where services are reduced; and rationing by termination, the ending of a service or intervention (Klein et al, 1996: 11-12). The different gatekeeping mechanisms used by all the teams will be compared to this typology of rationing in the remainder of this chapter.

The main mechanisms used by the generic/older person's teams to gatekeep access to assessments were: carrying out service specific assessments; requiring enquirers to be at risk; using service charges to dissuade enquirers; explicitly linking access to assessment to whether or not services could be provided.

Service-specific Assessments and Deflection

Although all the practitioners observed used a certain amount of jargon that was incomprehensible to many disabled people and carers, practitioners in the generic/older person's teams used it in a specific way that worked as a method of rationing access to assessments. Instead of referring to assessments by level ('initial', 'further' and 'full'), as was described in their procedures manual, computerized records system and the leaflets explaining the new community care arrangements that were available to the public, practitioners referred to different assessments as being service-specific. For example, assessments could be 'Home Care Assessments', 'Daycare Assessments' or 'Meals on Wheels Assessments'. This tendency was particularly ingrained in the Generic Team. The results of this approach can be seen in example 1 below:

> Example 1: The duty social worker received a telephone call from a community nurse about one of her patients, Mrs S. The duty social worker asked the nurse what service she thought Mrs S needed: the nurse didn't know, she thought the social worker should visit Mrs S to establish that. Mrs S had just had a knee operation and was having difficulty getting about. The nurse thought Mrs S needed a social work assessment. The duty social worker asked 'But what does that mean? Does she need home care, or what?' The nurse wasn't sure. The duty social worker decided that Mrs S needed a Home Care Assessment, and referred her to the home care manager for an assessment.

Not only was there no consideration of whether Mrs S had the right to an assessment, the practitioner in this case wanted the referrer to make a decision about the type of service Mrs S needed, to the extent of growing quite impatient with the nurse when she refused to make this judgement. How should the nurse, or anyone else referring someone for an assessment, know to ask for a 'Home Care Assessment'? In fact, anyone who was aware of the changes brought about by the NHSCCA would have expected to just ask for an assessment, as the nurse did, rather than expect it to be linked to a type of service. Example 1 also highlights how this use of jargon was compounded by the way in which people who were considered to need a 'Home Care Assessment' were referred to home care managers. In other words, they received an assessment from an in-house provider who would only consider their needs for one specific service: a practice directly in contradiction to the 'needs-led' ethos of the guidance accompanying the 1990 Act. Parker (1975) and Klein et al (1996) would call this a combination of rationing by deflection (making the request another person's or agencies' responsibility) and rationing by deterrence (making it difficult for applicants to access an assessment).

The study revealed that the practice of deflecting applicants to a service provider for an assessment was very common but limited to practitioners in the Generic Team. Local authority A did not appear to use provider assessments in this way, and it was impossible to establish whether the Deaf Team did so.

Risk, Need and Deterrence

Practitioners in the generic/older person's teams tended to only offer an assessment to people they considered to be at risk: they were supported in this by their formal procedures (see above). However, they did not usually think that people who had live-in spouses or relatives were at risk: they assumed that these spouses or relatives were full-time carers, whether or not they considered themselves to be carers, or were willing to take on that role. Someone who was receiving family care was considered not to need statutory services. Example 2 shows the results of this approach:

> Example 2: Mr and Mrs T's daughter had phoned the duty social worker the day before to ask for an assessment for her father, who was refusing to wash or care for himself and causing Mrs T some distress. Mrs T was very frail and registered disabled herself. Yesterday's duty social worker had interpreted this request as Mrs T needing some advice on how

to care for Mr T, so had referred them to a local carer's voluntary agency. Miss T did not think this sufficient, and felt she was being fobbed off. Today's duty social worker asked in some detail about the type and level of personal care that Mrs T provided for her husband. The duty social worker's view was that as Mr T had been discharged from hospital without any home care, Mrs T must be caring for him and his needs couldn't be that urgent. He thought the daughter's attitude was unhelpful: she was being 'bolshy and insisting on legal rights and throwing her weight around'.

In example 2, the duty social worker made the decision that Mrs T was coping as Mr T's carer without ever speaking to Mrs T herself, or visiting the family to ascertain what care Mrs T provided and what Mr T needed. He referred the family to a home care manager for a Home Care Assessment, but made it clear to the researcher that this was really only to keep the daughter quiet.

The fact that Mr T's daughter came back the next day, irate and convinced that she had been fobbed off, is an indication that not only is this type of rationing often likely to be unsuccessful, it would appear from the evidence that it is also likely to backfire and end up placing front-line practitioners in even more stressful encounters with enquirers than would otherwise have been the case. Klein et al (1996) refer to this type of rationing as rationing by deterrence: making it difficult for people to gain access to an official or assessment in the first place, discouraging people from applying for scare resources or services. However, as example 2 shows, it is a form of rationing that is very difficult for practitioners, disabled people and their families, and is not always particularly successful.

The need to show yourself to be at risk in order to access or be prioritised for an assessment could mean that when resources were tight you might fail to access an assessment altogether. Example 3 shows this happening in the Generic Team:

Example 3: During the period of the study, local authority B experienced a staffing crisis which meant that the Generic Team would lose one practitioner to another team without a replacement. When this issue was raised in a team meeting, the practitioners were worried that this would add to the waiting time for assessments for those people considered to be at a lower risk. One practitioner was concerned that this would create an unmanageable 'waiting list' for assessments. Her manager replied that this would not be the case - people at a lower risk would simply not receive an assessment at all. He justified this by saying there was no point making people wait for assessments if it is likely that there will be no money to offer them any services.

For those people considered to be at a lower risk, this rule would appear to function as Klein et al's (1996) rationing by denial: denying that the needs presented are urgent or sufficient enough to warrant consideration. It is also of interest that the manager and practitioners considered themselves able to make a judgement about a person's risk without carrying out an assessment at all.

Using Service Charges and Denial

Although charging service users for social care services is not a new development, the Griffiths report preceeding the community care changes made it clear that a central tenet of the changes was the assumption that people who could afford to do so should make a contribution to the cost of any social care services they received (Griffiths, 1988). The 1983 Health and Social Services and Social Security Adjudications Act gives local authorities the discretion to set charges for domiciliary services (unlike residential care, the charges for which are set nationally). One study of local authority charging policies found that not only did the basis and level of charges vary considerably between local authorities, but that how individual practitioners interpret their local authorities rules sometimes varied as well (Baldwin and Lunt, 1996). A complementary study of disabled people's experiences of services charges found that the charges were considered to be confusing, ill-explained, bore little relationship to actual services received, and were a cause for some people of significant financial worry (Chetwynd et al, 1996). Nevertheless, service charges are now used so widely by local authorities that they are considered a necessary part of authorities' finances (John, 1998) and a significant and unremovable barrier to effective collaboration between health and social care (because NHS services are largely free at the point of delivery) (Rummery and Glendinning, 1999).

Both the local authorities in this study charged service users for services either provided or commissioned by them. This affected all the teams apart from the Blind Team who, as a charitable organisation, were able to offer many of their services and equipment free of charge to service users. However, the fieldwork notes only revealed examples of the generic/older person's teams using service charges as a gatekeeping mechanism. Example 4 highlights this gatekeeping:

> Example 4: The duty social worker received a telephone call from Mrs A, who suffered from agoraphobia. She lived with her daughter who was in full-time education. Mrs A wanted someone to do her shopping and collect her pension on the days she was too afraid to go out. The duty social worker asked how many hours a day was Mrs A's daughter in college? Could the daughter not collect Mrs A's benefits on another day? The social worker tried to persuade Mrs A that as her daughter was 18 she could manage to collect her benefits for her, but Mrs A insisted she wanted someone else to do it. Finally, the duty social worker pointed out that if social services got her a home carer to collect her benefits she would have to pay for it: it would be much better for Mrs A's daughter to do it. Mrs A wanted information about the charges: the duty social worker said it was impossible to say without doing an assessment of what she would need, but asked Mrs A to think about why she would want to pay for a service that her daughter could provide for free.

As in example 2, the duty social worker is assuming that Mrs A's daughter is willing and able to provide the service, and that Mrs A is willing to let her daughter collect her money for her. It was clear from the encounter, and from remarks made to the researcher after the encounter (that visiting Mrs A or putting in a service would 'enforce her dependency') that the duty social worker was unwilling to carry out an assessment of Mrs A's needs. Introducing the idea of service charges at the outset thus seemed designed to dissuade Mrs A from pressing for an assessment, and the study showed that this was not an uncommon occurrence. Parker (1975) and Klein et al (1996) would see this as a combination of rationing by denial (denying that the need presented is genuine) and rationing by deterrence (deterring applicants from pushing for an assessment by making it clear that they will have to pay service charges).

'But We Don't Ration Assessments!'

During the course of the research, I was curious as to why only the generic/older person's teams had developed mechanisms for gatekeeping access to assessments: it appeared to me that they were rationing access to assessments as a way of managing the demand for services and resources. However, when I put this to the practitioners in the Generic Team during a feedback discussion, they were shocked. They maintained that they did not 'ration access to assessments': indeed the idea that any part of their role involved rationing was anathema to them. It went against their view of themselves as professional practitioners carrying out needs-led assessments.

On reflection the idea that only the generic/older person's team rationed access to assessments is misleading. All the teams operated a system of rationing by deflection: enquirers who did not fall within the client group, or whose needs appeared on first presentation to be related to health, benefits or housing were deflected to the relevant agencies. The study showed several occasion on which enquirers returning for an assessment, or where it was obvious that applicants had been re-referred by the relevant agencies when it became apparent they might have social care needs. Similarly, the view that only the practitioners in the generic/older person's team attempted to manage demand for services through rationing is misleading. All the practitioners used their professional status and their role in defining people's needs to ration access to services through the assessment process. The following section will explore this type of rationing in more detail.

Professional Gatekeeping Access to Services

As discussed above, the role that practitioners play in gatekeeping access to community care services is not in itself incompatible with the notion of disabled people's citizenship rights. However, how practitioners make decisions about need, particularly in how they interpret the way in which disabled people present their own needs, is obviously a crucial part of the assessment process. There are two elements to this issue that fall within the citizenship perspective adopted in this book: firstly, who, within the assessment process, do practitioners consider to be 'competent members of society' (Turner, 1993a) when gathering information about disabled and people's needs; secondly, how do the decisions made by practitioners affect disabled people's 'minimally curtailed social participation' (Doyal and Gough, 1991)? The first will be explored further in the remainder of this chapter; the second will be answered by the evidence presented by disabled people and their families and friends in chapters five and six.

Values, Models of Disability and 'Competent Informants'

There appeared to be a relationship between the model of disability used by practitioners in each team type, and the person considered to be the key 'competent' informant on need during the assessment process. The generic/older person's teams and the hospital team appeared to be working with a medical or individual model of disability, in which a person's impairment or illness, or their failure to adjust to that impairment/illness, are viewed as being the locus of a disabled person's problems. The result of working with a medical model of disability is clearly shown in example 5:

> Example 5: A practitioner returned from an assessment visit to discuss the results. Her client wanted to learn to play squash or tennis, but because of her medical condition she cannot stand up or feel the floor. The social worker and her supervisor felt that her desire to learn squash or tennis was unrealistic: the supervisor thought it was the result of the client failing to adjust to her lost mobility.

In fact, the local sports facility offered coaching in both wheelchair tennis and a form of wheelchair raquetball (very similar to squash). However, because the social worker's overwhelming consideration was to help her client come to terms with her lost mobility, all the needs and wishes the client presented her with were viewed from that perspective. The social worker felt that her professional status gave her view of the 'unrealistic' nature of her clients needs and wishes greater legitimacy: the social worker was the more 'competent informant' on need than the client.

Practitioners in the Hospital Team were particularly likely to use health workers as 'competent informants', giving their views on an applicants needs greater legitimacy than the applicants'. Example 6 illustrates this:

> Example 6: Mrs K was an Asian woman in hospital with a tumour under her arm. It was pressing on the nerves in her arm making it very difficult for her to use the arm. Mrs K wanted help when she went home with getting washed and dressed, particularly washing her hair, as her husband worked away from home a lot and her daughters provided unreliable help. The practitioner checked with the ward nurse, who felt that Mrs K's tumour wasn't that big and that Mrs K was overly concerned about some numbness. The practitioner told Mrs K

she would have to check the availability of services before anything else: Mrs K had been discharged before this was done.

Although it should not be suggested that the practitioner in example 6 was deliberately using delaying tactics to avoid having to offer Mrs K a service, she relied on the nurse's judgement of the urgency and level of Mrs K's need rather than being guided by how necessary and urgent Mrs K herself felt she needed the service.

'Citizen-the-Carer' Versus 'Citizen-the-User'

One of the most challenging, and revealing, aspects of the way practitioners made decisions about need was the relative weight they assigned to the information given by and the views of carers and users. Biggs (1994) characterises this phenomenon as the 'community care triangle': he describes three scenarios which may occur when worker, user and carer disagree on need. In the 'life task collusion' scenario, the worker and carer 'collude', because of similar experiences and outlooks, to exclude the views of the user. In the 'family solidarity' scenario the user and carer collude to exclude the worker and protect the family unit against outsiders. In the 'heroic defence' scenario the user is supported by the worker in excluding the carer from decisions about need.

The evidence from this study suggests that while Biggs' scenarios ring true, the decision made about need and who the practitioner considers to be the 'competent informer' are more complex and less static than the three scenarios would suggest. Who was considered to be the 'competent informant' varied not only according to the type of team in which practitioners worked, but also according to whether a potential service user was older and considered to be at risk.

Practitioners in the generic/older persons teams and the hospital teams tended to view carers as the 'competent informants', to a greater or lesser degree excluding the disabled person from decisions about needs and services. The results of this approach are shown in example 7:

Example 7: Mr B was an older man who was in hospital following a collapse due to over-medication. He was still feeling a bit confused when the assessment took place. His wife asked the practitioner (from the generic team) if Mr B could have a bath when he went to day care. The practitioner told her there was a waiting list for that service (known as 'tea 'n' tub'). Mr B pointed out that there was a bath at home - why could he not use that? Mrs B said that she couldn't bath Mr B at home without a walk-in bath. An auxiliary nurse present at the assessment said that the nurse couldn't get Mr M into a bath either. The practitioner, auxiliary nurse and Mrs B all agreed that Mr B would have to go on the waiting list for the 'tea 'n' tub' session. Mr B protested that this was a waste with a 'perfectly good bath at home'. His protests were put down to his confusion and ignored.

The practitioner failed to consider other ways of bathing Mr B that could be compatible with his wish to be bathed at home, such as a hoist into the bath or using two home carers to lift him into the bath. Mrs B's views and experiences were paramount: she was the competent informer in this case.

The practice of colluding with 'citizen-the-carer' as opposed to 'citizen-the-user' is supported by the normative core of community care of supporting informal carers to carry on caring, and thus save the cost of having to provide formal care (see previous chapter). Although in this case it meant the provision of a service (the 'tea 'n' tub session) that was a cheaper service than the possible alternatives that would have enabled Mr B to have a bath in his own home, and the service offered met Mrs B's needs. This is one reason why Morris (1997) asserts that the ethos of community care is incompatible with an ethos of independent living, or (to use the citizenship framework) the ethos of viewing disabled people as citizens, i.e. 'competent members of society'. This 'citizen-the-carer' approach adopted by practitioners in the generic/older person's teams, and the hospital team had the effect of prioritising the carers' needs, as is shown in example 8:

Example 8: Mr W had been going into respite care, which hehated. He disliked the food and objected to having to receive help with personal care from strangers. He also objected to paying for the residential respite when he had such a miserable time. However Mrs W found caring for him very hard work. She felt he was too demanding and had unrealistic expectations of respite care. She badly needed the break that respite care gave her. Mr W disagreed with his wife's view that caring for him was hard work. The practitioner assessing Mrs W persuaded him to carry on using respite care to give his wife a break. The practitioner felt it was important to support Mrs W in this way to prevent 'carer breakdown'.

However, it was possible for assertive disabled people to ensure that their views and definitions of their needs took priority over the view presented by carers. As example 9 shows, this could result in carers unwillingly taking on the responsibility to provide care:

> Example 9: Mrs S was in hospital with pneumonia. Her stepdaughter had requested the assessment, saying that she could not cope with caring for Mrs S. Mrs S was adamant that going into respite care would involve 'sitting around with a load of old women' which she did not want to do. Mrs S was also adamant that she did not want to accept domiciliary help, which she claimed would involve paying 'a young girl to come and watch my telly'. Mrs S's stepdaughter did the washing, cleaning and shopping for Mrs S and did not feel she could cope any more - there was much tension between the stepdaughter and Mrs S during the assessment. As the practitioner and researcher left, Mrs S's stepdaughter followed them and tearfully exclaimed 'you see what I have to put up with? It's too hard, it's too bloody hard!'. The practitioner explained that she could not put in services against Mrs S's will, but declined to try and persuade Mrs S to accept help.

During the course of the fieldwork upon which this chapter is based, the 1995 Carer's Recognition (and Services) Act had not yet been implemented. This gave carers the right to a separate assessment of their own needs. Without this protection, it was difficult for some practitioners to adopt an overtly 'citizen-the-carer' approach. This had two repercussions for such unwilling carers. Firstly, they were not considered to be the most 'competent' to assess the disabled person's needs, and secondly, their own needs, particularly their right to 'minimally curtailed social participation' (Doyal and Gough, 1991) were therefore not considered fully within the assessment process. Therefore if primacy was given to protecting the citizenship status (in terms of being considered the most 'competent' to decide on needs AND therefore accessing services designed to meet those needs and aid 'minimally curtailed social participation') of disabled people, the corresponding citizenship status of carers could be threatened, because they could find themselves unwillingly taking on extra caring duties that could curtail their social participation.

Practitioners in the specialist teams tended to treat disabled people as 'competent informants' and to feed information from carers and other sources through the lens of the disabled person's judgement. This could also place additional strains on carers, as example 10 shows:

> Example 10: Mrs C was a blind woman living on her own who
> had been referred for an assessment by her daughter, who
> travelled to see her nearly every day to do her cleaning,
> washing and leave her cooked meals. Her daughter was tired
> out by all the travelling and wanted Mrs C to consider moving
> to sheltered accommodation nearer her own village - she was
> worried about her mother's risk living on her own so far away.
> However, Mrs C was reluctant to leave the house she had lived
> in all her life. The practitioner agreed with Mrs C - she felt it
> was up to Mrs C to decide what level of risk it was acceptable
> for her to take in deciding to remain in her own home. Mrs C's
> daughter felt she could not abandon her mother, so had to
> continue with the travelling.

The practitioner (working in the Blind Team) in example 10
obviously felt that Mrs C was the most competent informer, compared to her
daughter, and so adopted what I call the 'citizen-the-user' approach to
assessment. This meant that a) the disabled person was considered the most
competent to assess their needs and b) that the provision of services was
thus geared to enabling them to participate in society in a minimally
curtailed way. This was not always the case. Even practitioners in the
specialist teams could abandon their commitment to the 'citizen-the-user'
and the fieldwork notes that this happened most often when they were faced
with an older disabled person whom they considered to be at risk, and not
able to make a competent judgement of that risk. Example 11 (where the
practitioner was also working in the Blind Team) contrasts sharply with
example 10:

> Example 11: Mr B was an older man with poor vision and
> mobility problems. He had asked to see the practitioner
> because he wanted an extra rail put in his bathroom. The
> practitioner examined the bathroom and said he was not happy
> about Mr B's safety in there. Mr B thought his safety could be
> improved by an extra rail but he didn't want any more help
> than that. He particularly did not want a home care assistant, as
> he would have to pay for that and he was worried about his
> money. The practitioner asserted that he was unhappy with Mr
> B's level of risk and he wanted to bring in his two sons to the
> assessment before proceeding. Mr B was unwilling to give the

practitioner his sons' telephone numbers - he didn't want the practitioner to bother them at work and he was unhappy with the thought that they would worry about him. The practitioner refused to continue with the assessment until Mr B agreed to let the practitioner contact his sons.

Not only was the practitioner in example 11 overriding Mr B's wishes and adopting the 'citizen-as-carer' approach, where the 'carer' was considered more 'competent' to judge Mr B's needs than himself (and it was by no means clear that Mr B's sons were doing any 'caring' work for him), the practitioner considered that his professional status put him in a better position to judge Mr B's risk than Mr B himself. This echoes Cheetham's (1993) concerns that a level of professional intervention is needed to decide on risk and need. Clearly, practitioners often found it difficult to balance the accounts of need presented to them, and where their judgement differed from that of the disabled person they would look for other informants they considered to be competent - Biggs (1994) would call this 'life task collusion', where the practitioner and carer collude because of their similar positions. In balancing who was considered the most competent it would appear that practitioners colluded with whoever in the assessment process presented them with information that reaffirmed their own judgement. However, this had the effect that the only real 'competent informant' in example 11 was the practitioner himself, because the sons, the potential 'carers', were absent from the assessment process at that stage and not really providing any information. Perhaps this approach is an example of a 'citizen-the-practitioner' approach, where it is the practitioner above all who is considered 'competent' to assess need?

Summary

The evidence presented in this chapter suggests that whether or not a disabled person could access an assessment, and thus be sure that their civil and social rights were protected, was dependant on the values and ethos of the type of team she was approaching. There appears to be some inequity in citizenship rights, in that younger disabled people, those with sensory impairments and those in hospital appear to be accessing assessments with greater ease than older disabled people living in the community. The implications of this ageist barrier to citizenship will be explored further in the next chapter.

The evidence presented in this chapter also suggests that practitioners will treat disabled people and carers differently as competent informers on a disabled person's needs, depending not only on the values and ethos of their team type, but also on how assertive a disabled person is, and whether they are judged by the practitioner to be a competent judge of their own level of risk. To an outside observer there appears to be no rhyme or reason to these decisions. Mrs C, in example 10, looked to the researcher to be much frailer and more at risk than Mr B, in example 11. Yet Mrs C was judged to be competent to assess her own level of risk and need, and Mr B was not. The bipartite construction of informants as either 'citizen-the-carer' or 'citizen-the-user' was also problematic for disabled people and their families, as is explored further in chapter six.

5 Negotiating Barriers in the Dark? Accessing Assessments

As was discussed in chapter four, for many practitioners and managers disabled people's civil right to access an assessment was not what drove the decisions they made about who should access an assessment. Assuming far greater importance was the need to manage demand for services by rationing access to assessments, using a variety of managerial and bureaucratic gatekeeping mechanisms described in chapter four. This chapter will address the question of the effect of accessing a community care assessment on the citizenship status of disabled people and their families, particularly on their civil right to enter the arena of negotiating access to their social rights.

This chapter will explore what it felt like to attempt to access a community care assessment. The evidence suggests that people experienced accessing a community care assessment in one of three ways: either as something that was imposed upon them (through being set in motion by someone else either with or without their knowledge); as a process of negotiating the barriers to assessment; or as a process that failed to culminate in what people recognised as an arena in which to negotiate their needs. This chapter will therefore explore the issue of what happens when your 'civil' right to an assessment is 'imposed' on you, what happens when you have to negotiate access to your civil rights, and what happens when you fail to assert your civil right to an assessment, exploring what each of those dimensions mean for the citizenship status of disabled people and their families.

As I was interviewing disabled people and their families it became obvious that hardly anyone who was interviewed was aware of the meaning of the word 'assessment' or that it bore any relationship to their experiences. This is not surprising: Baldock and Ungerson (1993) found similar problems although they put it down to the forgetfulness of old age. Although problems of recall are often an issue in research of this kind (Tulle-Winton, 1995), as very few of the interviewees had any trouble recalling other aspects of the process, it would appear that the problem was that the word 'assessment' fits

70

more with the jargonised world of the practitioner than with the experiences of potential service users. However, nearly all the interviewees appeared to have a similar definition of what the researcher meant by an assessment. They all recognised the idea of an 'arena of negotiating need': a space in which needs were discussed and negotiated with practitioners. This chapter will therefore discuss how disabled people and their families attempted to negotiate access to that space, and whether their civil rights were protected or threatened by the process.

Imposed Access

For some people, access to an assessment did not feel like something that had been negotiated or sought by themselves. It felt like something imposed upon them by an external system or person. This is not to say that the process was necessarily experienced negatively by these people: rather it was a process that was not under their control, that they did not fully understand or participate in. They sometimes welcomed the unsought intervention of the practitioner, although this intervention was experienced by some people as unnecessarily intrusive and wasteful of their time and energy.

These people fell into three main categories: those that had accessed an assessment in hospital; those who were referred by someone else, usually a family member, friend or neighbour who was concerned about them; and those who had entered into the formal process of being registered blind or partially sighted. The experience of these three groups was qualitatively very different, and they are discussed separately below.

Hospital

Several people had accessed a community care assessment while they were in hospital. For some this was linked to the way in which the hospital nurses perceived their needs, as Mrs Welling, an older woman living on her own, explained to me:

> Q: When you were in hospital the last time did you ask to speak to a social worker?
> Mrs W: No, the nurses said I needed the social worker.
> Q: Why did they think you needed one?
> Mrs W: Because I couldn't look after myself and I needed help.

And when I came home I had help mornings and evenings and weekends too, morning and evening.

Although Mrs Welling understood that the nurses had instigated her assessment, her memory of the actual assessment was less clear:

Q: How did the meeting with the social worker go?

Mrs W: I can't tell you about that because it's all so vague. She came and told me she was a social worker and that she would visit me at home. That's all I can remember because a lot of it in hospital I'm still very vague about. There are days that I can't remember.

This confusion about what happened during the assessment was not confined to Mrs Welling. Several other people had difficulty remembering what was actually discussed during an assessment encounter because it appeared to happen out of the blue, without any prompting from themselves or any warning. Mrs Dashwood's experience shows one of the explanations for this confusion. She was an older woman who was staying with her daughter at the time of the interview, and her daughter explained to me:

Miss D: The [social workers] were very helpful. They floated in, said who they were and took the information verbally, they didn't write anything down, and then went out again and we didn't hear anything else. By then you'd forgotten their names, so you didn't know who to get back to. The ones who were the most helpful were the people who gave a card because whatever happened to you could always refer to that. But the social workers didn't give cards. The occupational therapist gave us her telephone number and her name written on a piece of paper.

For the social workers in the hospital team it made no sense to give patients a card with their name on it, as they acted 'interchangeably' as part of the duty team. However, this lack of information about how to access a social worker was problematic for many patients. As they did not instigate the assessment, and were often not given any warning about when it would take place, they were unprepared for what was involved and often did not think of any questions or about their needs until after the social worker had left. Mrs Dashwood was clear about what she thought the solution to this problem was:

Mrs D: They should leave a card with their name on and phone number so that we can contact them if we need them. But they don't, we don't know who they are, they just walk into the hospital, just say I'm so and so, first name usually, and that's as far as they get. You don't know why they are there, they just wander in and ask you questions and wander out again.

The other problem that Mrs Dashwood and her daughter pointed out was that in hospital, a patient is likely to be seen by any number of different health professionals, with different specialities, as well as social care practitioners and assessors such as social workers and occupational therapists:

Q: When you were in hospital did you talk to a social worker?

Mrs D: Yes, I talked to a - I think it was a social worker - well they asked me what I wanted, what I needed, two ladies. Who did we talk to [daughter], those two who came to see me?

Miss D: Well, we saw physiotherapists, an occupational therapist, who can round last week to do an assessment on mum for a stair lift, and we did speak to a couple of social workers, yes, when we really needed a bath rail. And what happens is, they give you their name when they come in, but my mum was so ill that you don't take the name in, what they really ought to do is give you a card with their name on, that would be ever such a help and then you would know who you could refer back to when you've made a request...I think there are too many doing the same thing. Not all of them - it's a bit of a mix up remembering which is an occupational therapist, which is a physiotherapist and which is a social worker.

Given that someone in hospital is, by definition, likely to be feeling unwell, it is hardly surprising that patients found it difficult to keep track of which professional had spoken to them about what. The nature of people's needs and lack of knowledge about which services were offered by which agency meant that they did not delineate their needs into 'health' and 'social' care needs, and they did not understand the limitations that social care practitioners operated within. Mrs Todd, an older woman living with her husband and son, described her encounter with a practitioner in the hospital:

Mrs T: One of the nurses said who have you got at home? I said my husband. What can he do? I said he does what he can, he's had a stroke. But I said he does what he can, he makes himself very useful and helps me as much as he can, he always has done. So she said about the social services. So I said, well the only reason I'd like them is for someone to come and put the vacuum cleaner round, I can't do things like that - And they came to see me and she said, well what was it you required, and I said someone to put the vacuum cleaner round and do heavy jobs. Sorry, we can't do things like that, we only do shopping. I said, well, I've got a son, I've got a daughter, I've got at least six neighbours and they all do the shopping for me, so what you're offering me is no good to me.

Mrs Todd had not asked to see social services, she was asking how she could get her own self-defined needs met. However, the seemingly arbitrary division between what was and what was not provided by social services bewildered her. She pointed out that in her opinion 'Cleanliness in the house is obviously as important as getting the shopping done. If the house gets all filthy and horrible, well!' Mrs Todd also identified another problem with being assessed in hospital:

Mrs T: When you're in hospital they encourage you to move a couple or three days after the operation, even if you only go to the toilet. But if you want help, it's there, you've only got to call the nurses. I used to try and manage by myself. Actually you'll find when you're in hospital everyone in the ward will watch you, and if they think you're going to fall there's a shout goes up for the nurse.

Mrs Todd thought that this 'safety net' of constant surveillance in hospital could lead to people having no real idea of how they would manage at home without the safety net. Other people echoed this concern. They did not feel able to judge what sort of help they would need once they got home. The hospital environment felt at once protective and alien, and they were not sure if their mobility and safety would be the same at home. Yet the assessments often took place so quickly that people did not feel that they had the time to voice such fears, or to explore their needs in any depth. Mrs Dashwood's picture of practitioners 'floating' in to see them without any warning, and leaving no follow-up contact details or information was shared by other people assessed in hospital. Mrs Cotton, an older woman living with her husband, felt quite confused by the way the practitioners appeared to approach her 'out of the blue':

> Mrs C: They said 'we can come and get you up in the morning' - I mean, I can bath myself - 'we can get you up in the morning, get you a cup of tea, and come and put you to bed'. Well obviously, we didn't need that and 'we can bath you' well we didn't need anything like that, we can manage quite well... Well, I didn't understand - 'can you get yourself up in the morning, can you get yourself dressed?' - well I didn't want that sort of help!...I said to my sister, I don't know what [husband]'s playing at but the hospital seem to think we need help.... A lady came round and said 'What are you trying to get out of social services' I said 'nothing!' and she said 'what do you want?' I said I didn't want any of it.

Mrs Cotton felt quite affronted because she felt the approach had not come from her, yet she was being treated as though she was trying to 'get something out of' social services, something she felt the practitioner was hinting she was not entitled to. She said 'it's all been very strange. Not strange - I mean, nobody has been impolite to me, no-one, the lady was very forthright but she was truthful...It amazes me how this has escalated'. The arrival of my letter asking her for an interview further added to her distress: 'then out of the blue your letter came!'.

Mrs Cotton felt she had become part of a process that she had neither sought nor fully understood, which made her feel distressed and worried. Even the help that was offered to her was offered in such a way that she did not feel she was entitled to accept it, and it was made clear to her that she would have to pay for it. This she found a further affront: she was being offered services she had not sought, did not consider that she needed, and furthermore she was being asked to pay for them. The whole experience made her very unwilling to go back to social services, even though she knew her condition was likely to worsen and she might need more help in the future.

The next group of people reported different concerns: they had been 'referred' to social services by someone else while living in the community, and so felt they had entered into a process not entirely of their own volition.

'Being Referred'

Some people experienced a process of 'being referred' without their knowledge or permission outside of the hospital environment. Although they were warned of the practitioner's visit, they often did not fully understand the process that they had been entered into. Mr Kerr, a younger Deaf man, was referred to social services by his aunt:

> Mr K: My aunt told [social worker]- I don't know who told my aunt. Somebody told her, I don't know who, somebody in my family. [Social worker] came to see me last year for the first time...she talked about everything, about benefits...she helped me fill in the forms.

Although Mr Kerr was confused as to why the practitioner had originally come to see him (he thought it might be due to his aunt, or his attendance at a deaf club) he was clear that the help the practitioner offered him was welcome:

> Mr K: She helped me get Income Support then - Incapacity Benefit - in March we hope I'll get more money...this year [social worker] and someone from the Citizen's Advice Bureau came together to sort it out.

Mr Kerr had been left a letter with details of how to contact his practitioner, which he showed to me during the course of the interview when I asked if he had any other questions for the practitioner. He was also aware that he would probably meet the practitioner at the deaf club. While he did not fully understand the process of assessment, or why he was originally contacted by the practitioner, subsequent information given to him by the practitioner appears to have been sufficient to enable him to be able to contact her again.

Other people living in the community sometimes felt that the practitioner had been contacted by someone who wanted to 'prescribe' certain services for them. While they appreciated that this usually happened out of concern for their well-being, they did not always share that concern. Mrs White was an older woman living in sheltered accommodation who was referred to social services by her warden. She explained to me:

> Mrs W: I'm content enough here, you know. They worry about me not moving out of this room enough to go to the common room. Now, there's a concert on tonight with some dancers,

and the warden is going to come and take me down and they're worried a bit about me not getting out. They think I should get out a bit more and they did suggest a day centre...The warden thinks it would be a change for me. But whatever they do I shall just go, but if I don't like it I won't go. I'm happy enough to sit here, I can see what goes off and [the home care assistants] come and see me three times a day.

The warden obviously felt Mrs White may be lonely and needed more social contact with others, whereas Mrs White did not particularly feel the need to go to daycare. However, people who had been assessed in the community in this way did not report the same level of feeling rushed and unable to articulate their needs as did those who were assessed in hospital. In the community they were usually given notice of the assessment and were often given information about how to access a practitioner should they have further unanswered questions.

It cannot be said that either the group assessed in hospital or the group assessed following referral without their knowledge spoke of the experience to me in terms which might indicate they felt they had accessed a civil right. They did not feel that their status as 'competent members of society' had in any way altered, let alone improved: apart from a couple of people who were worried that they were now on a social services list and would therefore be monitored in some way without their approval, and were therefore in some way now considered to be less 'competent' than they had been prior to the process. To these people, it felt as though accessing an assessment was in some way a stigmatising process, rather than a right: they had been considered lacking in some way by either the hospital or by whoever had referred them in the community. This could in part be explained by the relatively low levels of information that these people had about the assessment process, and the way in which practitioners in the hospital and generic type teams did not treat the assessment as a civil right. The evidence discussed in chapter four would suggest that practitioners in these teams could in some cases act as though they believed that people entering into the assessment process were, by definition, less 'competent members of society' than those who were not considered to need local authority services or support.

The final group of people who experienced an assessment without having sought it themselves (or it having been sought by a carer on their behalf) were those that were registered blind or partially sighted. This group not only had a qualitatively very different experience to the previous two groups, but also experienced the process in terms of gaining status and accessing social rights. For this latter group the process of accessing an assessment, even though it was not at their own behest, was generally a process which protected their civil rights and facilitated the access to social rights which would enable their social participation.

'Being Registered'

In order to be registered blind or partially sighted in the UK, a consultant must assess the level of your eyesight and then inform your local social services department, who carry out the formal registration process. Within this study this process had been contracted out by local authority B to a county-wide charity for the blind, the Blind Team.

People who had experienced this process had not initiated it themselves (although several had originally approached their doctor with failing eyesight). Nevertheless, they felt much better prepared for the process than either the group assessed in hospital, or the group who were referred without their knowledge in the community. Mrs Leith, an older woman living alone who was partially sighted, explained:

> Mrs L: They came through the consultant at [hospital] or wherever it was they registered me as partially sighted. They came then. I had a letter first to say they were coming.

Because she had had notice that the practitioners were coming, and because she understood the link between the consultant's actions and the practitioners arriving, Mrs Leith felt quite prepared for the visit. She (like the other interviewees who had been registered blind or partially sighted) felt that the meeting with the practitioner had been very thorough and covered all her concerns. Mr Wishart, an older man living on his own who was registered blind, felt the registration process had gone well for him:

> Q: Did you have any questions when [practitioner] came out?
>
> Mr W: No, I didn't know much about it.
>
> Q: Did you know more about it when she had finished?
>
> Mr W: Yes I was a bit surprised.
>
> Q: What were you surprised about?
>
> Mr W: All the things they covered. I didn't expect a service like that. I'm the old fashioned sort and look after myself.
>
> Q: Did you think it was a bit intrusive?

Mr W: No, not really. I got used to it a bit when she was talking about different things. I know I couldn't see much, so any help I could get I didn't mind...Up until this I didn't know much about them but they seem very reasonable.

Several of the people in this group enthusiastically listed the equipment or training they had received from the blind team that had improved their lives:

Mrs A: [The practitioner] offered me a lot of help, he gave me a single cane, various things from the RNIB to write a letter, address and envelope, lots of things... he gave me what they call UV shades, very up to date, sunglasses to me, which help, and a talking clock which is very useful.

Mrs C: [The practitioner] started off by giving me a white stick and because I don't hear very well she put some red stuff round it...She organised Talking Books. I now get the tapes from [local library] and I have that [indicating brightly marked tape recorder] on which to play them because I can't see the knobs on the ordinary radio. I've got a watch, I've got a clock with a thing that goes under my pillow which vibrates if I can't hear the alarm.

Mrs H: They brought a talking clock and wrist watch for me, but my husband uses the wrist watch because he can't see a clock or a watch and I'm using his...and they brought a radio cassette player. They were very helpful. To me it was the end of the world. And they joined us up with the library and we get the Talking Newspapers.

Many of the people in this group described losing or having their sight circumscribed in similar terms to Mrs H: it was like 'the end of the world', a devastating and confusing experience. The practical assistance they were offered by the blind team was greatly valued precisely because it enabled them to maintain contact with the outside world, carry out tasks they had thought were impossible with their reduced sight, and to maintain a level of independence. In other words, the practical assistance offered throughout the assessment process enabled blind and partially sighted people to consider themselves 'competent members of society' (i.e. citizens) once more. They were able to engage in 'minimally curtailed social participation' and to be able to discharge what they perceived as the duties of citizenship. This theme will be explored further in the next chapter.

Being registered blind or partially sighted was also considered by people to confer certain benefits and a status worth having. Mrs Addison (the Mrs A above), an older partially sighted woman, explained some of the benefits:

Q: You said you wanted to be registered partially sighted. Why was that?

Mrs A: Well, it's not just the benefits, it is beneficial because you can get different concessions, shall we say. I'm going on holiday this week and you can get a discount coach card, you can get a disabled person's railcard, I can get free tapes from the library. It's recognisable. People have said: you look alright, why the white stick? But that white stick gives you the confidence to go.

Mrs Nott, an older partially sighted woman living on her own, was also clear about the benefits she gained from her registration:

Mrs N: My son-in-law went to the public library...the mobile library, they are very kind to me, because they know me from when I was sighted, and they said that they only carry a certain amount [of talking books] which I can understand. And he went to the public library in [local town] and they said, well, you'll have to pay for the [talking] books if you want them which was 69p each. Well, of course it runs up a bit, but she said if [consultant] certifies you as partially sighted you get them free...My son-in-law went to social services and told them I was registered partially sighted and they said, is she having all that's due to her...and he said well, no, my wife does all the shopping and taking her to the doctors or the hospital, and looks after her generally, and so they said well she's entitled to Invalidity Care Allowance.

Mrs Nott felt that receiving an additional financial benefit also aided her independence: she paid it to her daughter for the shopping and other help she was given. This had the effect of legitimising her accepting her daughter's help: 'I feel better about her doing things for me now. Because it all costs money, doesn't it, petrol'. She felt less of a burden on her daughter, and more of a 'competent member of society' (i.e. citizen), which she equated with being able to pay her way. Many of the people in this group reported feeling that the registration process unlocked benefits (not just cash) to which they felt entitled: it was a passport to receiving social rights. The fact that it was a formal process made it feel like a civil right, and hence there was not the stigma attached to accessing the registration process that was felt by some of the people in the previous two groups. This was reinforced in part by the practitioners in the Blind Team (and other specialist teams) who tended to treat the registration (and assessment) process as a civil right, and the accompanying services, equipment and training as social rights. One practitioner, in trying to persuade an older woman to accept the benefits of registration, said 'it's only what you are entitled to. If you don't take this up, the money and everything will only go back to the government to waste.' This sense of entitlement was echoed by people in this group far more often than in any other group.

The fieldwork notes reveal that practitioners in all teams offered benefits advice or referred applicants to welfare rights officers as part of a 'full' or 'comprehensive' assessment, particularly if applicants ending up receiving services (in part because benefits such as Attendance Allowance were taken into account when calculating service charges). People sometimes mentioned in interviews that their practitioner had helped them with applications for Attendance Allowance or Disability Living Allowance, but only people who had been assessed or registered by the Blind Team consistently spoke of this help in ways which I interpreted as being about accessing rights and as being without stigma. There was a definite link in the minds of this group between the formalised registration/assessment process and perceiving the accessing of assessments and services as a right.

For some people in this group the registration process gave them a status which legitimated their 'invisible' impairment to the world. Mrs Nott and Mrs Addison both mentioned this as an important factor of the registration process. Being able to carry a white stick meant that they did not have to explain why they found negotiating steps and curbs, or reading, difficult. Mrs Compton (the Mrs C above) said that 'If anyone asks why I've got red stuff on my white stick, I just tell them I kick, because that is what they put on horses' tails!' Being registered, and having some obvious sign of that registration such as a card or white stick, reduced the need for lengthy explanations: it gave people a legitimate status of being blind or partially sighted.

Negotiated Access

People who either attempted to access an assessment themselves in the community, or whose carers, family members and friends attempted to access one on their behalf, had very different experiences from that group of people on whom assessment was imposed. They reported having to negotiate a series of barriers, sometimes partially or wholly 'in the dark' about the location and significance of those barriers, before being able to gain access to an assessment.

Many practitioners would assert that they were gathering information on people's needs during the course of this barrier negotiation, and that people were therefore accessing an assessment earlier than they realised. However, as discussed previously, this made no sense to people who had been assessed. They understood the concept of an assessment as being akin to the 'arena of negotiation of need' described earlier. This meant nothing less than a face to face meeting with a practitioner. The various barriers experienced by this group of people, and the ways in which they sought to circumvent them, are discussed below.

Networks, Knowing the System and Using Third Parties

The initial barrier experienced by people was in gaining access to a practitioner. As one woman pointed out, social services have about 20 telephone numbers in the telephone directory: how do you know which one to call? This was of particular concern to those who were worried about telephone bills mounting up on a low income as they were passed around until they reached the correct department. (The issue of 'being passed around' is discussed in further depth below) As discussed previously, assessment systems often appeared to have been designed with the needs of managers and practitioners, rather than potential and actual service users, in mind. Accessibility for potential service users took a low priority, particularly if managers felt an overwhelming need to ration access to assessments as a way of managing demand for resources, as they did in the generic-type teams.

This access problem was exacerbated by the fact that most people, unless they had a history of contact with social services, were unaware of the duties and responsibilities of social services departments, and did not understand how their needs might fit in. For example, they could not necessarily distinguish between a 'health' and 'social' need (Twigg, 1997), or even articulate their needs in a way which would tally with the eligibility criteria and services provided or purchased by social services. In short, they did not necessarily know that their query should be dealt with by social services, or, given the differing organisational arrangements that were found even within just the two local authorities participating in this study, which branch of social services.

Many of the people referred to friends and acquaintances to try and 'stop up' some of the gaps in their knowledge about how to get help from social services. Some even made the initial approach to social services following advice from a friend or acquaintance, such as Mr Keswick, a younger man who did so following advice from a fellow patient in hospital. He and his wife explain:

> Mrs K: While you are in [hospital] there was another chap, very similar to you, wasn't there, who suggested that you got in touch with social services because he'd been in touch with them himself and was having various things to help him, wasn't he?

For Mr Keswick, what persuaded him to get in touch with social services was the fellow patient's assertion that he was entitled to help:

> Mr K: He said, we've been to work all our lives, so why shouldn't we get something if we're entitled to it, and I thought, well, yes. It was something I hadn't thought about before, and if I was entitled to something, OK, I might as well have a go.

A sense of entitlement, or of accessing a right, appeared to be more acceptable to many of the people than a sense of asking for help with needs. For some, a sense of entitlement was linked to their view of their own needs, as Mrs Anderson, an older woman staying with her daughter, articulates about wanting some money to pay her daughter:

> Mrs A: It's not just the money, it's the principle. Other people get it, why shouldn't I?...I think to myself, if you are entitled - other people get it, there's nothing wrong with them, they must know all the angles.

For Mrs Anderson, entitlement was about measuring her needs compared to other people who were receiving the sort of services, help and benefits which she considered that she needed. But as Mr Keswick's experience shows, accessing what you are entitled to (in this case a community care assessment) is not that simple:

Mr K: When I came out of hospital I rang the social services and she asked me what I wanted, on the phone actually, and I was a little bit put out I must admit. She was a nice girl, I met her afterwards, but she said 'What do you want?' and I said I didn't know what I wanted. And she tried to talk to me on the phone, and I thought that was impossible. I said 'I can't talk to you on the phone, I can't tell you what I want because I don't know what I want.' I said 'I want you to tell me what I'm entitled to and what I'm not entitled to. In other words, tell me all about it because I just don't know.' I said ' I can't tell you on the phone.' She was on about pull ups for the bath and things like that, and anyway eventually she arranged to come and see me and she was a very nice girl when she came.

Mr Keswick felt that it was not realistic to expect him to know what to ask for on his first approach to social services. He explained:

Mr K: The very first time I phoned up, when I asked the question, I don't know whether they expected me to know, I think that was the impression I got, that they expected me to know what I wanted, and I didn't, I hadn't got a clue...She wanted to know how I knew about social services. I said 'The bloke in the bed opposite'. And she said, did somebody see you in the hospital about it? I said 'No'. But she said somebody at the hospital should have seen me. But then again I never asked anybody at the hospital because I didn't know about it.

Mr Keswick has highlighted the dissonance between an assessment system designed to meet the needs of practitioners and managers, and one designed to meet the needs of potential service users. Firstly, the 'system' dictated that Mr Keswick 'should have' had an assessment in hospital. However, no-one thought to refer him to the hospital social work team, and he did not know enough about it to refer himself. Secondly, Mr Keswick did finally manage to access an assessment from the Generic Team. The practitioner he was talking to on the telephone would have considered the telephone call to be an assessment in itself. However, Mr Keswick did not consider a telephone conversation to be an adequate discussion of his needs: he did not feel as though he had entered 'the arena of negotiation of need' until he met the practitioner face to face. He described what he would change about the system and why a telephone assessment was unsatisfactory:

Mr K: I would...want her to come and see me, I wouldn't want to talk on the phone because you can't have a proper conversation on the phone, there's the bill for a start, and you can't have a proper conversation, not unless it's a short sharp answer you want. The things I wanted explaining - how can you spend half an hour on the phone explaining it? If you've got somebody in the house to talk to... then you've got all the time in the world to explain what you want or what you might need.

Some of the people in this group had had previous contact with social services, and were aware that 'inside knowledge' on the best way to approach them would improve their chances of securing access to an assessment. Mrs Guest, a younger blind woman who lived with her husband, had a long history of contact with social services. When she needed additional equipment, she contacted her local voluntary agency to find out the best route to social services (this happened to be the Blind Team). She explained:

Mrs G: I've been able to sort of get to know what I wanted from contacts I think more than anything...you learn to know [the system], I tend to find out more through dialogue with [Blind Team] more than anything...but I haven't seen a social worker in years.

Sometimes, people in this group were already receiving health or social care services, and found that using their service providers to access an assessment offered a quicker route than trying to contact a social worker themselves. Mrs Welling, an older woman living on her own, explained what she would do if she needed extra help:

Mrs W: I'd ring [number]

Q: And what would happen then?

Mrs W: I'd tell them I needed extra help, and they would speak to the home helps about my condition and if she thought I needed it, I would get it.

Q: So who's on that number, is it the social worker?

Mrs W: No. Home helps. You see, if you get in touch with the social worker you have to wait for her to come out and see you. If you go straight to the home helps' office it's quicker.

Although using this procedure meant that Mrs Welling was accessing a service provider assessment rather than a full community care assessment, she was adamant that the quicker service response she got was much more important to her than the more thorough, but delayed, assessment she would have accessed from a social worker. Other people found that mentioning a service provider by name when contacting social services sometimes seemed to 'quicken things up', particularly if they mentioned a health care provider such as a district nurse. One couple, Mr and Mrs Sheldon, were so incensed at how difficult it was to get through to the right person at social services to deal with their query (they wanted to access a Meals on Wheels service) that they threatened to involve their local councillors. Very few correspondents went to those lengths to assert their civil right to an assessment, but there was considerable disquiet at how difficult it was to even get to speak to a practitioner on the telephone, let alone persuade one to visit for an assessment.

Timing of Assessments

As well as negotiating the barriers to assessment erected by practitioners and managers, this group of people highlighted their concerns that the timing of assessment was crucial. Assessments that happened too early (for example some of those that happened in hospital) did not enable people to have an accurate idea of their needs. A more common complaint was that it took people so long to try and access an assessment that their needs deteriorated, or were unnecessarily higher by the time the assessment happened. Being able to access an assessment was therefore not just about gaining access to the 'arena of negotiating need' with a practitioner, it was about gaining timely access to that arena.

Mrs Douglas was a younger woman who had a hip operation in a private hospital and was then sent home without any help. She describes the frustrating time she had trying to get help from her social services department:

> Mrs D: As soon as I came out [of hospital] I rang [the social worker in the Older Person's Team]. His very first words were 'oh well, we'll have to send somebody out to assess you', so I said 'well I want some help tomorrow morning, I'm on my own'...he said 'oh well we've got to come out and assess you and see what you need.' I said 'well I need someone to help get me out of bed for a start'. Then he said 'they'll be here in a

couple of days' and I said 'that's no good to me' because it was coming up the Bank Holiday week.

Mrs Douglas was then passed around various offices (see below), which further delayed her accessing an assessment. This delay led to considerable distress, as she describes:

> Mrs D: I'd got this sickness and diarrhoea, and I felt terrible, in fact my daughter had the doctor in to me...in the end I got through to [Younger Person's Team], to be quite honest I was quite crude. I asked if I'd got to lie in a shitten bed all over the holiday, because I was at the end of my tether...
>
> Q: If you had the head of social services here...what would you say?
>
> Mrs D: Well the first thing I would ask them to improve would be to get their act together and act when people want it. That's the main thing...Initially from the very beginning - if we'd had the help from the beginning we wouldn't have any problem.

While few people felt that the delay in accessing an assessment led to a risk that they would have to lie in excreta-soaked sheets, as Mrs Douglas graphically describes, delays were a common complaint. Many people had to wait for several weeks before seeing a practitioner, a few had to wait for up to a year. People reported that delays were particularly long when there was a need for equipment, or when people were attempting to access an assessment from one of the specialist-type teams. The fieldwork notes revealed that these teams coped with the fact that they offered an assessment to everyone who approached them by operating a waiting-list, although it was not possible given the methodology to check data on delays between referral and receiving services so I cannot say how long a typical delay was. Those people who experienced delays which caused them concern tended to blame these delays on what they considered to be poor management and lack of staff. Mrs Gate, an older woman who waited a long time for help from the Blind Team for herself and her husband, who was blind and Deaf, explained:

> Mrs G: The doctor referred me, he sent the letter in October and I got an answer in February, they said they could have someone come out to assess [husband] in August. They came out in October. [The rehabilitation officer] had to have someone bring her, she said 'I've just had 65 referrals given to

me from [local social services] where somebody has been off
on maternity leave. 65 in one week.

Mrs Isher was also concerned at the year long delay it took her to get
an assessment for her Deaf son from the Deaf Team, which she also put
down to a lack of staff and poor management. Poor management was also
blamed for the way in which some people found delays in accessing an
assessment exacerbated by being passed around between different teams
and branches of social services.

In some respects, from a citizenship perspective a delay in accessing
an assessment is not a threat per se to disabled people's citizenship status.
After all, all people eventually did access an assessment and their civil
rights were thus protected. However, as the discussion below highlights, the
assessment itself was only really of worth to people because it was the arena
of negotiating needs and access to services to meet those needs - it was the
outcome of the assessment, and whether it unlocked access to services and
support that enabled disabled people to maintain their 'minimally curtailed
social participation' that was important to them. A delay in accessing an
assessment therefore meant a delay in accessing services, which could mean
that for a period of time disabled people and their families could experience
what felt to them like avoidable and distressing levels of social exclusion.

Being Passed Around

Social services departments are large, complex organisations and no two
seem to be organised in exactly the same way. Most separate out their child
protection work from work with adults. A further organisational divide is
the way in which some departments operate a 'single entry point' system,
whereas others have numerous possible entry points. Some departments
operate 'specialist' disability, sensory impairment and older person's teams,
some have 'generic' teams covering some, or all of the above. Nearly all
seperate mental health services from other adults services, and some also
separate learning disability services. Added to that, several local authorities
(including the two which took part in this study) have reorganised the
organisation of their services following the implementation of the
NHSCCA, and some have changed shape yet again following the local
government reorganisation of recent years and the creation of some unitary
authorities.

All in all, the myriad organisational possibilities are confusing even
to people with several years of experience with social services. It is almost
inevitable that a novice to the system will attempt to access what they need

the 'wrong' way at first. Some people who had attempted to enter the system the 'wrong' way found themselves rebuffed. Most of them found that they were 'passed around' the system from one branch or team to another, with very little explanation of what was happening and why.

Although the design of this study did not allow me to get the practitioners' perspectives of the same events, by coincidence I happened to be carrying out observations in the Younger Person's Team during the period that Mrs Douglas (above) was trying to access an assessment. The observation notes reveal that there had been some confusion initially over Mrs Douglas' age: was she 64 (in which case she was the responsibility of the Younger Person's Team) or 65 (the Older Person's Team)? Matters were then complicated by the initial failure to realise that she had received her hip operation in an out-of-county private hospital: if she had received her treatment on the NHS at the local hospital she would have been assessed by the Hospital Team. Several fruitless days passed while an attempt was made to track down her (non-existent) records at the Hospital Team until one practitioner realised the mistake. The issue was further confused by the revelation that Mrs Douglas was the main carer to her husband who was an ongoing client of one of local authority A's specialist sensory impairment teams (not featured in this study). Further delays were experienced when the manager of the Younger Person's Team tried to persuade the manager of the relevant specialist team that it was his responsibility to carry out Mrs Douglas's assessment. There were additional pressures because this episode took place during August, when all of the teams concerned had staff shortages because of annual leave. Finally the Younger Person's Team accepted responsibility for Mrs Douglas' referral and a practitioner was sent to assess her needs.

Mrs Douglas describes her experience in being 'passed around' thus:

Mrs D: There are lots of people far worse off than me, but the downfall as far as social services is that the left hand doesn't know what the right hand is doing. You've got no communication between one department and another...I was passed from [Older Person's Team] to another social services department, God knows where it was...They gave me two numbers to ring because I came home on the Monday and I rang [practitioner from Older Person's Team]. When he hadn't come by Wednesday I rang again and a girl said he wasn't there and put me through to a different department. I got an answer machine so I left a message that I wanted them to ring me because I needed some extra help.

The distressing results of this delay for Mrs Douglas are discussed above. Mr Patterson, an older man living alone, and Paul, his neighbour, had some ideas on how this type of confusion could be avoided:

> Q: So it would have been better to have more information?
>
> Paul: Oh yes, then he'd know where he stood instead of guessing all the time. Could I apply for this, maybe I'm entitled to this. If it was all down in a booklet.
>
> Q: With phone numbers?
>
> Paul: Yes, free phone numbers, because of [Mr Patterson] being a pensioner. It would be ideal, then he could ring up, I could ring up. I rang up a few times for [Mr Patterson] because he tends to get a bit muddled up on the phone...
>
> Q: Did you have to deal with all that phoning up yourself?
>
> Paul: Yes. Find out the numbers and what departments.
>
> Q: Did you get passed to different departments?
>
> Paul: Yes, until I got the right one. Wrong department!

People found delays in accessing an assessment distressing and often felt that a timely intervention would have prevented their needs from escalating. People described how their families and friends often had to take on providing quite high levels of care, sometimes unwillingly, while these inter-agency and inter-departmental disputes and negotiations were sorted out. Mrs Douglas' granddaughter had to stay with her and provide a level of intimate personal care that Mrs Douglas felt uncomfortable with. She was also adamant that, had it not been the school holidays, her granddaughter would have been unable to care for her and she would have been left to lie in excreta-soaked sheets by the time that social services had finished 'passing the buck'. Delays of this kind were considered unacceptable by many of the people in this group, who felt that they were being made to suffer needlessly due to social services' incompetence and lack of organisation. They felt that the state (in the shape of social services) was reneging on its duties to them as citizens.

As was discussed above, this group's experiences of delayed access to assessment, while worrying and distressing for them, do not pose that much of a threat to their civil rights, as all of them eventually managed to access an assessment, to gain entry to the 'arena of negotiation of need'. The threat to their citizenship status came primarily from the threat to their social rights and the curtailment of their social participation that people experienced as a result of the delay in accessing services. However, the barriers they experienced were in many cases incomprehensible to them. They were not a part of the formal procedures laid out in information leaflets, or if they were people did not have access to that information. They could not therefore challenge those barriers.

Barred Access

Some people found it almost impossible to gain access to their definition of an assessment (a face-to-face meeting with a practitioner to negotiate need), despite the fact that, all the of the people in this study did access some level of community care assessment as defined by social services practitioners and managers. The barriers described and discussed in chapter four proved to be insurmountable for them. While the prime concern for the previous group of people was the timing of assessments, and the delays caused by being passed around the system, the main concern for this group of people was being able to gain access to an assessment at all.

Service-specific Assessments

The first hurdle that many people found insurmountable was that they did not know when attempting to access an assessment which particular services were available, and which they thought they might need. This proved a particular difficulty when people were dealing with teams such as the Generic Team, who operated a quasi-formal system of service-specific assessments (see chapter four, section on bureaucratic gatekeeping).

Mr Keswick (see above examples) encountered this problem when he contacted the Generic Team after his stay in hospital. He was asked over the telephone which service he wanted. As he explained:

> Mr K:...she [practitioner] said 'What do you want?' and I said I didn't know what I wanted...I want you to tell me what I'm entitled to and what I'm not entitled to. In other words tell me all about it because I just don't know.

As discussed above, the fact that Mr Keswick did not know what he wanted (i.e. he was not aware of the patterns of services available in his area) delayed his access to what he conceived as an assessment (i.e. a face to face meeting with a practitioner). He experienced this delay as a bar to his access to an assessment, and felt that had he not been adamant about pursuing the matter, he would never had accessed an assessment at all.

Although Mr Keswick's lack of knowledge was shared by many

people, some people had a very clear idea of the services they wanted to receive. Mr and Mrs Wilson, an older couple who both accessed assessments, did so because they wanted a Meals on Wheels service and access to a service known as Ring and Ride (a transport service for disabled people). They were interested in other services, particularly home helps, but when they realised that the home helps could not give them help with housework maintained that they would prefer to make their own arrangements. Mrs Loughton, an older woman living on her own, similarly contacted the social services department because she wanted a specific service: in her case it was a home help to help her with preparing food.

Mrs Cavanaugh, who was caring for her husband at home, was adamant that she would only approach social services for a specific service and was not interested in anything else. She and her husband explain:

Mrs C: I never bothered with social [services] or nothing, people said I was silly at the time, but...I was terrified, you know -

Mr C: We never look for anything -

Mrs C: There is only one thing bothers me now, we have no phone, and someone said that the social [services] would help you...but we're managing.

For the Cavanaughs, it was important to show that they could manage without help, and they did not want the stigma of receiving help or services from social services. This stigma would be lessened for them if they requested one specific service, rather than made a general request for help. From their description of their circumstances, there were several services locally that they probably would have been assessed as needing, had they wished to pursue these options with their practitioner. But they valued not having to accept these services: they felt that their independence was heightened by their right to refuse anything but very specific help.

Although the reluctance to accept services was shared by other people (see the next chapter for a fuller discussion of this) not all of them were as aware of the availability of services, and which services they specifically wanted, as the Cavanaughs, Wilsons, and Mrs Loughton did. This was only likely to prove a bar to accessing an assessment if they were attempting to access one from the Generic Team, and to a lesser extent the Older Person's Team (who used Home Care Managers to carry out 'home care assessments'). None of the other teams used service-specific assessments in this way.

As the following section will show, there was a dissonance between what was considered by interviewees and practitioners to constitute an assessment. The practice of carrying out assessments over the telephone was considered to be a barrier to accessing an assessment by some interviewees.

Telephone Assessments

The practice of carrying out assessments of need over the telephone is most graphically illustrated using Mr Keswick's experience (see above). He attempted to access an assessment by telephoning a practitioner working in the Generic Team and found, to his surprise, that he was expected to discuss his needs with her over the telephone. This was not acceptable to Mr Keswick. He did not know which services were available: he wanted a full discussion with the practitioner about what he was 'entitled' to. He did not wish to have his telephone bill mount up. He found it difficult to have lengthy telephone conversations because they made him breathless, exacerbating his medical condition.

Mr Keswick wanted access to an 'arena of negotiation of need', and he interpreted this arena as being nothing less than a face to face meeting with a practitioner. Indeed, when he did finally persuade the practitioner to visit him, the discussion was satisfactory and met his demands for the 'arena'. As he explained:

> Mr K: [the practitioner] put me in the picture about all aspects of it, I think. She was here quite a while, and she did put us in the picture quite well about all the different aspects, but at the time I hadn't got a clue. I explained to her I didn't know about these things and I'm not after anything either, I said if I'm not entitled to anything so be it, I said, but if I am, OK, I'll have it if I can.

Mr Keswick interpreted the practitioners' questions over the telephone about what he wanted not as requests to define his needs in terms of the services available, but as a hint that he may be seen as a 'scrounger' and asking for things he was not 'entitled' to. He interpreted the assessment process as being about finding out what he was 'entitled to', i.e. finding out about his civil and social rights. He did not consider it to be possible to carry out that process over the telephone.

His practitioner, on the other hand, interpreted the assessment process as being a way to match applicants to the available services, hence her questions over the telephone. Although this was distressing and unacceptable to Mr Keswick, it was not the overt threat to his citizenship status that service-specific assessments were. If she were challenged formally, the practitioner could legitimately argue that the telephone conversation did itself constitute an assessment of Mr Keswick's needs. Although this poses concerns about the balance of power to define what constitutes access to the 'arena of negotiation of need' that is the assessment, from a citizenship perspective the fact that Mr Keswick was not actually barred from accessing an assessment means that his civil rights were not in fact under threat.

It could be argued that an assessment that is not recognised as such by both parties, particularly by the applicant who is in any case in a much less powerful position to understand, let alone dictate the form of the process, is not a meaningful assessment. One way in which telephone assessments could be interpreted as a threat to Mr Keswick's civil rights is that he, personally, appeared to have no say in whether or not the assessment was carried out over the telephone. The scope of this study did not allow for any examination of whether the use of processes like this were subject to consultation with services users, but I suspect (given that telephone assessments were not used by the specialist teams in that local authority) that this was a bureaucratic, rather than managerial process, probably designed to save money by reducing the need for practitioners to travel out to applicants' homes. As was argued in chapter four the use of bureaucratic gatekeeping is a threat to disabled people's citizenship because the bureaucratic processes employed are not clear and open to challenge using judicial processes.

However, it could be argued that a more substantial threat to people' civil rights could be found within the formal, managerial gatekeeping mechanisms such as the eligibility criteria for who should access an assessment. These criteria appeared to offer a significant barrier to assessment for carers attempting to access an assessment on behalf of disabled applicants. The most substantial threat to disabled people's citizenship status from the use of processes such as telephone assessments appears to be the threat to their social rights which resulted from them being unable to enter an arena where they could negotiate their needs in a way that was meaningful to them.

Being a Carer

In those teams which did not acknowledge disabled people's right to access an assessment (and thus operated eligibility criteria for who could access an assessment as well as for who could access services), having, or being a carer per se appeared to be a reason to be denied access to an assessment. This is illustrated most clearly by the example of Mrs Rackham, a younger woman caring for her husband, who was living at home. He had multiple sclerosis. She had been trying for some time to get help with caring for her husband, and found that she could not access an assessment or any services or support. It was only when she herself was taken ill, and was suddenly unable to carry on caring for him, that they received any response from their local social services department (the Generic Team).

She explains:

> Mrs R: I have had one heart attack, some time ago, and that was the only reason we got any help then, wasn't it. When I went into hospital he was left and all the social services were around then, but until then nobody had bothered to come and see us at all.

Inadvertently, through removing her care because she was in hospital, her husband became eligible for an assessment, whereas previously it had been impossible for Mrs Rackham to get anyone to visit them. She describes her fruitless quest to get help:

> Mrs R: Up until then there was nothing. Until I had that heart attack, and then of course they were all here, but until then - I'd rung up to ask about the bath - and months and months went by and they didn't even reply or make an appointment, and we were going away on holiday in the May, and I phoned them in case they were planning - and she said, oh no, I didn't know anything about it. And still nothing came, and then I had the heart attack in the December, and they were here.

Mrs Rackham felt that having to bathe her husband and cope with everything herself was a significant factor in the deterioration of her health that led to the heart attack. When they finally managed to access an assessment (due to Mr Rackham being without a carer, and thus eligible for one) Mr and Mrs Rackham felt slightly overwhelmed by the help that was offered:

> Mrs R: We never heard anything until I landed in hospital and then they were here, and they've supplied a bath seat, they supplied a stool, they've supplied a walking frame, a grab rail.

> They are supposed to be doing something about the front
> porch, because it's a step down... And of course they asked if
> we wanted any help to come in for putting him to bed or to get
> him up or things like that, and we don't actually need that.

The civil right to an assessment is not, according to the legislation or guidance, contingent upon the disabled person not having a live-in carer. However, as was discussed in chapter four the Generic Team did not formally recognise disabled people's right to access an assessment in their eligibility criteria. The practitioners and manager in this team seemed unaware of that right, and so did nothing in their formal procedures, gatekeeping or day to day practice to enforce that right. Consequently, they had eligibility criteria to help practitioners decide who should access an assessment, and these were based around whether or not the applicant was considered to be at risk. According to these eligibility criteria, having a live-in carer was considered to be proof that someone was not at risk, so Mrs Rackham found it impossible to access an assessment for her husband. At the time the study took place the Carer's Act (giving carers the right to an assessment) had not come into service, so it is difficult to say whether Mrs Rackham would have had any more luck attempting to access an assessment from the Generic Team on her own behalf. The fieldwork notes reveal several examples of applicants for assessments being deterred because they were, or seemed to have, carers, and this was echoed by some people, but the relatively low numbers of 'carers' who were not themselves disabled who took part in interviews made it difficult to assess how common an experience this was.

However, Mrs Rackham's experience is a clear indication that where managers and practitioners are unaware of, or unwilling to support, disabled people's right to access an assessment, disabled people's civil and social rights, and hence their citizenship status, is threatened. Had she known about her husband's right to access an assessment Mrs Rackham would have been able to challenge the practitioner's original decision that he was not eligible for an assessment. Of course, the delay incumbent in challenging decisions judicially would probably mean that she still would have experienced a delay in accessing an assessment, and her health would still have been put at risk in the meantime by the pressure of caring for her husband.

Threats to the Civil Right to an Assessment

The evidence presented in this chapter suggests that there are significant threats to disabled people's civil right to access an assessment. These threats are posed mainly by the managerial and bureaucratic gatekeeping mechanisms employed by social services managers and practitioners to manage access to community care assessments as a way of managing demand for services and resources. In practice, these threats display themselves in such processes as the maintenance of the inaccessibility of social services departments, the timing of assessment being designed to meet practitioners rather than applicants' needs, the way applicants are passed around the system, carrying out service-specific and telephone assessments, and making someone with a live-in carer ineligible for an assessment. They are significant for disabled people's citizenship status because they threaten both their civil rights (the right to access an assessment) and their social rights (the right to services to meet their needs). If disabled people are barred from gaining access to the arena in which to negotiate their needs (the assessment) they are barred from accessing full citizenship.

The following chapter will explore what happened to the citizenship status of disabled people and their families when they did enter the arena of negotiation of need, the assessment itself.

6 Being a 'Competent Member' of the Community: Services and Social Participation

The previous chapter explored the issue of citizenship in terms of disabled people's right to access an assessment, and the various ways in which that right can be undermined or even denied by social services' managerial and bureaucratic practices. In this chapter, the assessment itself is conceived as one of the 'various practices' which define a citizen as a 'competent member of society' (Turner, 1993a). It will explore the ways in which various people are constituted as 'competent members of society' during the process of needs negotiation which takes place between disabled people, 'carers' and practitioners. It addresses the question of how disabled people and their families experience the assessment as a way of negotiating their needs and access to services and support to meet those needs: in other words, how they access their social rights.

When viewed within the framework of the assessment process, there are two elements to being considered a 'competent member of society'. The first, discussed in the following section entitled Negotiating Need, concerns the way in which needs are negotiated and who is considered to be a 'competent' assessor of need. Within this chapter, the competing claims of the various participants to be considered the most 'competent' to assess the disabled person's needs builds on the analysis begun in chapter four of the 'citizen-the-worker' versus the 'citizen-the-user' scenarios. The discussion includes an analysis of the role of the practitioner in the process which might point towards a solution to the competing claims for citizenship: the scenario of the practitioner as a 'co-citizen', which will be further explored in chapter seven.

The second element of citizenship concerns the way in which services, ostensibly designed to meet needs, either permit or hamper an individual's inclusion within society as a competent member, or how far services aid or hinder a person's ability to engage in 'minimally curtailed social participation' (Doyal and Gough, 1991). What effect does the outcome of the assessment process have on the citizenship status of disabled people and their families? This is discussed in the section entitled Social Participation and the implications of the results presented in this chapter are explored further in the latter half of chapter seven.

Negotiating Need

Earlier chapters highlighted how disabled people and their families recognised the concept of an assessment (even if they did not recognise the actual term 'assessment') as being the arena in which need was negotiated. They understood the nature of an assessor's gatekeeping function, and thus that their own view of their needs could not simply be accepted resulting in instant access to the services of their choice. Indeed, as many people were unaware of the service options available, they would not have been able to articulate their service package of choice without the practitioner's assistance. The respondents understood the assessment as being a process by which their access to services was negotiated in accordance with how the assessor perceived their needs.

'Citizen-the-Worker' Versus 'Citizen-the-User'

Some of the respondents in the sample felt very strongly that their competency to assess their own needs had been discounted by the practitioner during the assessment process. Mrs Edgington had disagreed with her practitioner over whether she needed extra equipment. She had attempted to appeal to the practitioner's manager with no success. She pointed out the problems that occurred when she and her practitioner disagreed over her needs:

> Mrs E: I mean, who are people going to believe, her or me? They're going to believe her, aren't they? What leg have I got to stand on?...you ask her for any help...she's not interested.

Although Mrs Edgington went on to express dissatisfaction with her care providers as well, her point illustrates the problems that can arise when there is conflict between people being assessed and those doing the assessing over need. The practitioner is placed in the position of being an 'expert' on the disabled person's needs, a position which Cheetham (1993) and others endorse. There are two functional reasons for this position of expertise. The first is that the practitioner is acting as a gatekeeper to a limited pool of resources, and when she accepts that a 'need' really is a need, it most likely translates into a demand upon those resources. Cheetham's question 'do users' and carers' wishes for a service equal a need for it?' (Cheetham, 1993: 164) is particularly salient, given the gatekeeping role. Of the two local authorities which participated in this study, the awareness of the gatekeeping role was shown most clearly by practitioners in local authority B, who worked with explicit cash limits on the service packages they could offer applicants.

However, a second functional reason for the practitioner being constituted as the expert on need within the assessment is the practitioner's professional status. The practitioners in this study were all either qualified social workers, social work assistants or rehabilitation officers, all of whom undergo some kind of training giving them the professional status necessary to undertake an assessing role for the local authority. This, combined with the fact that the practitioners are party to information on the local authority's eligibility criteria and hence know what will be accepted as 'need' in a way that most of the respondents did not, places the practitioner in a very powerful position. This power imbalance caused the interviewees some concern - it was not so much that they were being denied access to services (although this concerned them as well) but that instead of saying that a service was unavailable practitioners would disagree that the service was actually needed. In some cases, such as Mrs Edgington's, interviewees felt that the practitioner treated them as though they were stupid and lacked knowledge of their own needs, or to use the citizenship epistemology, that they were not competent to assess their needs. When Mrs Edgington was asked what she would change about social services, she replied:

> Mrs E: [they should] try not to make you out to be stupid...
> [they] try to belittle you...Sometimes people think if you can't
> remember anything, they try to make you out to be stupid.
> Even [Mrs E's favourite practitioner] does.

Mrs Edgington had had a series of disagreements with her practitioner over whether she needed different equipment and some new accommodation (she was fifty years old, and in very sheltered housing with residents who were mostly over the age of seventy). However, because she was in a type of accommodation that was scarce and expensive, her practitioner was unwilling to try and find her alternative housing. Mrs

Edgington describes one particularly frustrating conversation with her practitioner:

> Mrs E: I said I wanted to be moved from here, I said I wanted my own place. And she said 'oh you can't do that' because I hadn't been here long enough, and then she said I wasn't high on the priority list like I had been before and I would have to wait ages. You see, I'm the youngest here, I'd love a place of my own. I know I'd have to have carers coming in and I'd be able to have a dog.

It would appear that Mrs Edgington's practitioner was using her position of being a professional expert to judge that Mrs Edgington's need for new accommodation was not urgent. The practitioner made it clear that such accommodation was scarce, but what really caused Mrs Edgington concern was the way the practitioner had tried to persuade her that she did not need new accommodation. This resulted in Mrs Edgington feeling that the most 'competent member of society' able to assess Mrs Edgington's needs was the practitioner, not Mrs Edgington herself.

This problem was made particularly acute by the lack of information that people felt they had about the availability of and eligibility criteria for services in their area. Mr Keswick experienced this when his practitioner expected him to be aware of the range of services available and to know himself whether his needs fitted in with the eligibility criteria of those services. As was quoted in the previous chapter:

> Mr K: I rang the social services and she asked me what I wanted on the phone actually, and I was a little bit put out I must admit. She was a nice girl, I met her afterwards, but she said what do you want and I said I didn't know what I wanted.

Mr Keswick did not feel he had the necessary information to act as a 'competent' judge of his needs in these circumstances, and was surprised and displeased to find that he was expected to do so.

Other people reported other difficulties with the power imbalance between themselves and their practitioners. Mrs Harrison, an older woman living on her own, found that she was having to overstate some of her needs in order to access the help she felt she needed. This made her feel uncomfortable, as she says:

> Mrs H: It doesn't do to be truthful, and I know it sounds awful, but the doctor said I'd got to have...this TENS machine switched on...My neighbour switched it on this morning but... I have to have it regularly.

She deliberately did not tell the practitioner that her neighbour occasionally came by to offer her help and switch on her TENS (pain relieving) machine, because she knew that the practitioner would then say she didn't need domiciliary care assistants to come in and do it for her. Mrs Harrison's assessment of her needs was that she needed to be able to rely on someone coming in regularly (something she did not feel her neighbour could provide), but she felt that her practitioner's assessment of her needs would find that her needs had been met by her neighbour. Other people reported similar feelings of unease at what they felt was sometimes having to underplay the level of irregular informal support they received from friends and family because they felt they needed more reliable, formal services but suspected that practitioners would assess the irregular informal support they received as adequate. They reported that this unease would have been reduced had they felt that practitioners would have trusted their view that the help they were receiving was not adequate (or, to use the citizenship epistemology, that they were competent in judging the level of their needs). As Ellis (1993) and others have found, this discrepancy in the power to define need is one of the core problems of the assessment system for disabled people.

Whether or not practitioners considered respondents to be 'competent' assessors of their own needs was made irrelevant when encounters were so brief that respondents did not feel they were given an opportunity to articulate their needs. Mrs Hargreaves, a fifty year old woman caring for her two school-age children, felt that practitioners:

> Mrs H:...like everyone else, they've lost contact with the world, they are too busy doing this and that, and saving this and that, they haven't got time for people.

Mrs Hargreaves felt strongly that not only was the practitioner acting as a gatekeeper to resources, but that the practitioner was also a gatekeeper to her own resources of time, particularly the time it would take to explore the issue of needs thoroughly with Mrs Hargreaves. She said she understood the pressures that practitioners were under, but pointed out the problems associated with not being given adequate time to articulate her needs:

Mrs H: If they refuse you [help] it's another rejection, another set back, and your esteem gets even lower then. It is like being mentally ill and you go to get help and they tell you to go away and come back later. I know there aren't the resources and the people...they try their best...what pittance they get, and they're dedicated - It's money problems all the time, they're only allowed to do so much with limited funds, basically it comes down to money.

Mrs Hargreaves felt that being set up against the 'immovable barrier' of lack of money, and lack of time to discuss her needs properly with the practitioner, had made it much harder for her to cope with both her own needs, and the needs of her children. She felt that once she had been told there was no money to provide the service she considered she needed, there was no way to appeal against the practitioner's judgement. She also felt that the practitioner's overwhelming agenda of saving money, and her view that her own professional status put her in a better position to judge Mrs Hargreaves' needs than Mrs Hargreaves herself, limited the sort of help she was offered:

Mrs H: The [hospital] nurse said 'When you go home you know you should not go home and jump into work and that, you won't be able to.' And I thought, 'Well, who's going to do it if I don't do it?' There's nobody else here to do it, you can't expect kids to be adults, because they're not adults, they're kids...[the social worker] was more interested in me going to [name of hostel] to help someone else, to be honest with you. Because I went to [name of hostel], it's like a women's hostel, and they were fantastic, they were marvellous, and they asked me to go voluntary, one day a week, and I couldn't, because I've got all my problems and someone else with the same problems as mine putting it all on me, I couldn't take that!... All she was interested in was me ringing up [name of hostel] and getting in there and getting it done.

Mrs Hargreaves' practitioner obviously had her reasons for encouraging Mrs Hargreaves to do some voluntary work with the local hostel, but that completely missed the point, as far as Mrs Hargreaves was concerned. She felt she had real, practical needs, and that the practitioner was neither acknowledging those needs, nor helping her find an acceptable way of meeting those needs. The practitioner presented Mrs Hargreaves with her opinion that she did not meet the criteria for services, and Mrs Hargreaves felt there was no appealing against that decision:

> Mrs H: I had the idea that maybe they could find some way of helping me, but they couldn't. I didn't meet the criteria... because I could make a cup of tea and I could get the dinner on, and I could get dressed myself, so I didn't qualify. They said the only thing they could do for me was shopping, and that was no good, I could get a neighbour to do some shopping...

Mrs Hargreaves felt that the system, and the practitioner's role within it, did not bear any relation to her own needs:

> Mrs H: I was knocked back by 'we can't help you, you don't fall into any category', I mean what category have you got to fall into to get some help? I didn't fall into any category. It's the system, I can't fight the system. I haven't got the energy, I've got to pool my energy to look after me and the kids.

She wanted help looking after her children, but the only help available would be for her children to be taken into care, which she did not want. Mrs Hargreaves was clear that she felt the practitioner's status as a social worker added to her problems:

> Mrs H: I think the problem is with social workers...I don't like social workers, to be quite honest, nobody does, do they, because it is a stigma which goes back years ago...I think it sticks with you. Those at [the hostel] are not social workers, they're health people, volunteers...but they helped. I don't like social workers as such because I think they're nosy, and you've got to answer to them...the difference between being nosy, and dropping in and seeing if you're alright, it's different.... when I was in [the hostel] it was great because I got support. It's all to do with support.

Mrs Hargreaves felt that the hostel workers offered her help in a pragmatic way that did not create a hierarchy of competency. They were not gatekeeping access to resources and had no reason to have knowledge about services, procedures and eligibility criteria that put them in a more powerful position than her. Her view of her practitioner, on the other hand, was that she did not see Mrs Hargreaves as a competent citizen, but as a person demanding unavailable services who should really be going out and helping others as a way of taking her mind off her own problems. Mrs Hargreaves' relationship to her practitioner could be constituted within the assessment process as one characterised by the 'citizen-the-worker' approach discussed previously. In contrast, her relationship to the hostel workers, who were also welfare state workers, was perceived by her as being much more equal - the workers were her 'co-citizens' rather than being considered more 'competent' members of society than herself.

The practitioners' power to decide what constitutes a valid need made some respondents feel that their judgement was unvalued. Mrs Todd lived with her husband, who had recently had a stroke, and her son, who had mental health problems. She was in hospital following a heart attack when she discussed with her practitioner the option of getting some extra help around the house. She had no success, and when asked if she would change anything about social services replied:

> Mrs T: I would certainly ask why we're not allowed this help when it is essential...I would approach them and say 'Well, why can't I have the essential things done that I need in the house. I would push it...I think...it's essential that these jobs should be done. Anybody who's really disabled they need someone to perhaps clean the house up, do the washing and the shopping. I think those are the three essential things that need to be done.

But Mrs Todd's practitioner did not agree with her that these things were 'essential' (in part probably because housework was a service no longer offered by the in-house provider in the area). Mrs Todd also felt that her needs as a carer of her son and husband were also ignored by the practitioner:

> Mrs T: Well, I do honestly think that carers of disabled people do need a break which they don't seem to be able to get by having anyone else come in, to give the carer a break. To me, there doesn't seem to be any communication there. In my instance I was worn out looking after [husband] [before he recovered], a carer is on 24 hours a day, and one does get very tired, and I think you should be able to go to the social services and say do you think you could find someone to look after my husband while I have a week or a fortnight's break.

Mrs Todd felt that the practitioner was only willing to discuss her own personal care needs, and unable to recognise that she also had caring responsibilities. This separation of 'user' and 'carer' has been discussed previously, but it did cause some of our respondents difficulties in having their needs heard by practitioners. It sometimes increased the gulf between what respondents considered to be 'essential' needs, and what were considered to be needs by their practitioners.

Users Abdicating from Citizenship

Some people found themselves in a position where they did not really want to be considered a 'competent member of society' but felt they needed the practitioner to take that role on their behalf. This was particularly the case for people who had been assessed in hospital, where they felt too ill or tired to be able to articulate their needs. Mr Cotton described the assessment thus:

> Mr C: It was a bit confusing...I wasn't in any condition to ask any questions, I'd just had an operation and to me it was a bit of an ordeal really.

Several other people echoed Mr Cotton's view that having to discuss their needs was an 'ordeal' that they could well do without, on top of the ordeal of being ill and in hospital. However, none of these interviewees reported that practitioners appeared to be willing to take over the 'competent member of society' role and decide for them whether or not they needed any help. It would appear that practitioners were only willing to see themselves as 'more competent' to assess need when there was a disagreement between themselves and respondents. They were less willing to undertake this role when respondents considered themselves unable to perform the 'competency' role and make an assessment of their own needs.

Practitioners as 'Co-Citizens'

Only one group of people felt that the practitioners' role as a more 'competent' assessor of their needs than themselves was justified. Interviewees who had been registered blind or partially sighted by a blind or partially sighted practitioner valued the 'co-citizenship' status, in a sense of being considered an equally 'competent member of society', that this conferred on their relationship with their practitioner. Several of these respondents described how their practitioners brought their attention to new, practical suggestions for services or equipment that they had not been aware of, and which increased their independence greatly. Mrs Guest, who was registered blind and had had several years experience of social services, claimed that this element of the practitioners' expertise was overlooked when managers reorganised social services teams:

> Mrs G: Only [practitioners] who are specialised in it are any help. I don't think it's the fact that they're not aware, it's just that they're not able to [meet blind people's needs] because they are having to cope with so many different things, like child abuse or battered wives...If they are forming teams... surely there could be somebody there who deals with the different aspects of it, because no one person can specialise in everything.

Other people who had been registered blind or partially sighted often echoed Mr and Mrs Douglas' view of one of their practitioners:

> Mrs D: [Practitioner] was blind herself, and she was trying to get him a home...
> Mr D: She's blind and a diabetic.
> Mrs D: She's got the same kidney condition as [Mr D], so she knew exactly what he needed. She said, if we look at a 'blind home', like the one locally, she didn't think that was going to be appropriate because it was all elderly blind people.

The view that practitioners 'knew exactly what was needed' because they themselves were blind or partially sighted was echoed by nearly all the people who had been registered blind or partially sighted. These interviewees described less of a sense of a 'power imbalance' between themselves and the practitioner, and more of a sense of the practitioner as a 'co-citizen'. A 'co-citizen' was a supportive friend or advisor who gave equal weight to their own versions of their needs, and offered services and equipment as practical aids, rather than as resources that needed to be gatekept. In a relationship characterised by the 'co-citizenship' approach, the practitioner's superior knowledge about the availability of services and equipment did not put them in the position of being 'citizen-the-worker', i.e. a more 'competent member of society' than the disabled person. Rather, the practitioner's knowledge was offered to the disabled person as an equally 'competent member of society' whose own knowledge about their needs and capabilities was balanced by the practitioner's knowledge of the availability of services and support.

The only other group of respondents who felt that practitioners had any particular skills or knowledge which put them in a better position to be a 'competent' judge of their needs than the respondents themselves were those who had had the chance to build up a trusting relationship over time with the practitioner. Mr Daniels was a fifty-two year old man with multiple sclerosis who had built up a trusting relationship with his practitioner (who was also disabled) over a number of years. He explains:

> Mr D: [The practitioner] knows my circumstances anyway, because when I was in the nursing home she got to know me quite well. I was going through the worst part of my life, my wife was divorcing me at the time and she had put me in the nursing home. It was such a traumatic couple of years that [practitioner] became quite involved.

The level of involvement described by Mr Daniels meant that he felt the practitioner shared information with him about social services procedures and eligibility criteria, reducing the 'power imbalance' between them. He explained how helpful she was when his condition worsened:

> Mr D: Since I came out of hospital after having septicaemia, I couldn't stand up at all, I couldn't put any weight on my legs at all, so [practitioner] upped the care...she just talked it over. But now apparently I've gone over the budget.
> Q: What does that mean?
> Mr D: It is costing social services more than they are allowed to spend on me. [Practitioner] came round and said 'You've gone over budget' so she put down for me to have the Independent Living Allowance which is what I am waiting for now...somebody from the Independent Living Fund has been around to the house and [practitioner] phoned me up a couple of weeks ago and said that she's been told by phone that I've been granted the Independent Living Fund...that would mean somebody to live with me for a fortnight so I would have somebody with me 24 hours a day...I'm quite keen on that actually.

Unlike many other respondents, Mr Daniels did not feel he had to argue with his practitioner over his needs: rather, he felt his practitioner was a supporting 'co-citizen' who understood his needs and was a valued broker of services on his behalf. His feelings were shared by some people who had not had such a long history of involvement with their practitioner, but who felt that practitioners had made some effort to address the power imbalance by sharing information with them. Many of the respondents who were blind and partially sighted had received accessible information about their assessment or registration, and felt free to call upon the practitioner for help and advice again. Other people also valued being given clear written information and being encouraged to contact the practitioner again after the assessment. They felt it went some way towards addressing the power imbalance of the assessment situation whereby they were expected to articulate (and sometimes campaign for) their needs within a time frame dictated by the workload of the practitioner.

The Powerful Position of 'Citizen-the-Worker'

The concerns expressed by the respondents in this section reveal some problems with the formulation of community care assessments that place practitioners in a much more powerful position to be the 'competent' assessors of need than disabled people themselves. 'Citizen-the-worker' appears to take precedence over 'citizen-the-user' in assessing need due to the practitioners' better knowledge of available services and eligibility criteria. This knowledge, and the practitioners' professional status, created a power imbalance between themselves and the disabled person, leaving interviewees feeling as though they were less 'competent' to assess their needs than the practitioner.

There were some actions which could be taken by practitioners to counteract this power imbalance. Practitioners' need to act as gatekeepers to limited resources could be much less of a problem for people if practitioners were disabled themselves, or had specialist training particularly in the social model of disability and disability awareness, and showed an ability to be 'co-citizens', exploring previously unknown service or equipment options with respondents. A sense of both parties being considered 'competent' assessors of need was engendered by practitioners who made the effort to act as supportive advocates rather than those who used their professional status to be more 'competent' assessors of need than respondents.

'Citizen-the-User' Versus 'Citizen-the-Carer'?

One aspect that I had wanted to explore was whether or not 'citizen-the-carer' took precedence as a 'competent' assessor of need over 'citizen-the-user'. The previous chapter explores some evidence for this from the observations of assessment encounters. However, this aspect was impossible to explore with interviewees because they did not recognise the delineation between 'users' and 'carers' in the same way that practitioners did. Many people had a complicated net of duties and relationships, some of which appeared to place them in a 'caring' role (such as Mrs Hargreaves with her children, and Mrs Todd with her husband and son) and some of which placed them in a role where they were receiving help or care (such as Mrs Todd from her husband and son). Mrs Douglas, in the previous chapter, is the clearest example of how unhelpful the categories of 'user' and 'carer' could be: she experienced delays in accessing an assessment which caused her significant hardship because practitioners could not decide which category she fitted into.

The failure to uncover a 'citizen-the-carer' situation from the interviews with respondents may also reflect the research methodology. Disabled people who took part in the interviews were invited to nominate a 'carer' to take part in the interviews, and disabled people and carers all opted to be interviewed together despite being offered the opportunity for separate interviews. It is unlikely therefore that disabled people would have nominated a person whom they considered to have a radically different outlook on the assessment process than they themselves did.

Social Participation

While the issue of negotiating need during the assessment process was a vital component of disabled people's citizenship, it should not be forgotten that the negotiation itself was only a part of the process of attaining, and maintaining citizenship. More importantly, the assessment itself was a route to accessing services and support which disabled people hoped would enable them to live their lives with 'minimally curtailed social participation' (Doyal and Gough, 1991) - the assessment was the passport to social rights. Some people articulated a view of services as being something they had a right to, such as Mr Keswick's often repeated assertion that:

> Mr K: If I'm not entitled to anything, so be it...but if I am, OK,
> I'll have it if I can.

However, being a citizen, a 'competent member of society', had much wider implications than receiving their entitlements. Many people were experiencing increasing impairment, either as the result of a sudden crisis in their health or as part of a deterioration of a long-term condition, such as arthritis. As such, they were finding it increasingly difficult to participate in society in the way that they chose: they felt that they were hindered in carrying out the public and private duties which they associated with citizenship, and they were suffering a curtailment to their 'social participation' (Doyal and Gough, 1991) that could be expressed as increasing social exclusion. Mrs Crompton described the social exclusion she experienced when her hearing and eyesight deteriorated:

> Mrs C: The worst thing of all was being in a room full of people and everybody's talking at the same time, and one person tries to talk to me, and I can't hear a word they say. I can't read any letters, I can't read anything.

This left Mrs Crompton feeling very isolated and unable to engage in social participation in the way that she considered to be acceptable. She characterised her isolation as:

> Mrs C: I've lost my independence...I can't write things, you see, neither can I collect my thoughts. I think it's old age, and most of my problem is not being able to see.

The reason Mrs Crompton and others wanted to access services was to enable them to attain, or maintain, a level of independence which would mean being able to engage in social participation which was commensurate, in their view, with an idea of 'active citizenship' (Mead, 1986; Lister, 1997), of being able to fulfil their duties to act as social beings as well as having their civil and social rights protected. They wanted to regain a sense of social inclusion by returning to being 'competent members of society' with the aid of services, help and equipment that they had to undergo assessments in order to access. In this book I have explored some of the issues involved in accessing an assessment, and the process of the assessment, in either undermining or supporting disabled people's citizenship, in terms of the protection or otherwise of their civil right to an assessment and the way in which they were construed by the practitioner as being a 'competent member of society' able to assess their own needs. The remainder of this chapter will explore the concerns expressed by disabled people about the way the provision of services, help and equipment could either help or hinder their citizenship and social participation - the impact accessing (or not) their social rights could have on their status as citizens.

Practical Assistance and the 'Disabled Citizen'

Where services (or more usually, aids and equipment) were appropriate and provided in a timely and affordable manner, many people reported with joy the positive difference they felt these made to their ability to participate in society. Earlier in this chapter the issue of assessors as 'co-citizens', offering practical assistance in a supportive way which did not exploit the inherent power imbalance in the assessment process, was explored. This approach was welcomed by interviewees, who found that their sense of being considered, and being enabled to act as, a 'competent member of society' was enhanced by encounters with such assessors. This was increased when the outcome of the assessment (whether it was aids, equipment, advice or services) was appropriate to their needs and added to their sense of independence (which people often articulated as a better sense of control over their environment and a correspondingly reduced sense of isolation and dependence on help from others that was sometimes inappropriate and not under the control of the disabled person themselves) (Brisenden, 1985, 1989).

A sense of their independence improving as a result of the outcome of an assessment was most often voiced by those people who had received aids, training and services as part of the process of being registered blind or partially sighted. Mrs Addison was registered blind and listed the equipment she had received and found helpful during the course of her registration:

> Mrs A: A visually impaired social worker came to see me and he offered me a lot of help, he gave me a single cane, various things from the RNIB to write a letter, to address an envelope, loads of things...he gave me what they call UV shades, very up to date, sunglasses to me, which help, and a talking clock which is very useful. And he offered me training with the long cane. I'd got the RNIB white stick which I was used to so I said I didn't feel I needed that, I felt I was used to the white stick, and...he said I could always come back to him if I felt I needed. I didn't need the white stick for support, as he called it, I just needed mobility training to basically get around.

Mrs Addison explained that being registered blind did not just get her access to aids and equipment which helped her, but also gave her a recognised status that circumvented the need to explain her impairment:

> Mrs A: It's recognisable. People have said, you look alright, why the white stick, you see they don't know what degree vision loss you've got.

Mrs Crompton was another respondent who valued the explanatory status of the white stick:

Mrs C: [The rehabilitation officer] started off by giving me a white stick and because I don't hear very well she put some red stuff around it. Now if anybody asks me why I've got red stuff on it, I tell them I kick, because that is what they put on horses' tails.

The desire to have a badge of identity as a blind person is echoed by the desire expressed by many of the respondents with mobility impairments to have a disabled badge or sticker for their car. Aside from the obvious practical benefits of easier parking, many respondents also voiced the opinion that a disabled badge would give them the status of a 'disabled citizen'. This was a person who, while a 'competent member of society', had both the legitimate claim to extra social rights (such as the ability to park closer to amenities) which would facilitate their independence and social participation (in this example, to do their own shopping) AND were excused some of the usual duties imposed on other citizens (such as parking in the usual spaces). Whether the aid to shopping was a white stick (to navigate the pavement) or a disabled badge (to be able to park and reach the shops), the important factor about the aid to the respondents was that it enabled their social participation by both announcing their impaired status, and helping overcome the impairment at the same time.

Mrs Addison described the increased sense of independence that resulted from her having the white stick and the mobility training:

Mrs A: That white stick gives you confidence to go... I've got the single cane that isn't much good to me... I used to feel very what I call vulnerable at first, because it can work two ways, can't it? If somebody walked behind me, I suppose when you're on your own, I don't know, but I don't feel like that now. I don't feel like that now, I feel more confident.

She explained how her increased confidence had led to her being able to participate in society in a way she was comfortable with, making the link between the confidence she felt as a result of using her white stick and her empowerment as a social being:

Mrs A: I've got that determination, anything I really want to do I go for it. When you find you can do it you get more and more confident. It's better than sitting at home feeling miserable, you're no good to yourself or anybody else...I go out and I get the sociability, shall I say...They offered me the choice to go and try the day centre and they explained that most of the people there are older than I am...they offered me the chance to try it and I did, and I am very glad I did, it got me out.

The status and practical help she received as an outcome of the assessment process enabled Mrs Addison to exercise choices in her social life, enabling her to participate in society in a way that reflected her own chosen identity as a citizen, rather than an imposed identity as an isolated dependent person. Much of the equipment available to people being registered blind or partially sighted was designed to foster this sense of independence, as Mrs Hoskins found:

Mrs H: They brought a talking clock and wrist watch for me... and they brought a radio cassette player. They were very helpful. To me it was the end of the world, but they've joined us up with the library and we get the Talking Newspapers. They're terribly helpful, we've got phone numbers and can contact them. We can't really fault them.

For Mrs Hoskins, being kept in touch with news was very important and as her eyesight failed she felt she was losing that. Being put in contact with services that kept her in touch with the news added to her sense of independence and social inclusion.

It was therefore possible for the assessment process to enhance disabled people's citizenship, by providing them access to aids, equipment, training and services that both declared their status as impaired, and offered practical assistance in overcoming that impairment. However, this enhancement of citizenship status relied on the aids, equipment, services and training being appropriate in terms of timing, quality and cost. Those respondents who were registered blind or partially sighted often received services, particularly equipment, free of charge because it was provided through the local branch of the Royal National Institute for the Blind. They also tended to receive the equipment quite quickly as part of the formal process of being registered (see chapters four and eight for a discussion on the importance of formalisation in the assessment process).

This experience is in contrast to the experience of the rest of interviewees who reported that their social participation was curtailed by the assessment outcome, usually by not receiving services they felt they needed, or by gaining access to services that they considered to be inappropriate because of their timing, quality or cost. People also raised the issue of the way the assessment process and outcome reduced their choices - particularly the choice to take risks.

Citizenship Denied? 'Citizen-the-Carer' and the Availability of Services

No-one in this study had the right to any particular services (see chapters two and three). Nevertheless, people often felt that they needed particular services, sometimes highlighted during the assessment process, and expressed dismay and dissatisfaction when it became apparent that these services were unavailable to them. Many interviewees discussed their need for services which would enable them to provide help and care for others. They often voiced the view that providing such help was part of their way of being a 'competent member of society' and fulfilling the duties of citizenship.

At the time the research took place the 1995 Carer's (Recognition and Services) Act, which gave carers a right to an assessment of their own needs, had not yet been implemented and there was no particular recognition by either of the local authorities who took part in the research of the need to provide services to support carers, even when those carers were themselves disabled. Assessments, and both the provision of and funding for services, was based around individual service users and their needs, usually for personal care services. There was no provision of services specifically to support carers: in fact, as discussed earlier in this chapter and in chapter five, assessment systems and protocols often could not allow for the fact that many disabled people had caring responsibilities.

The example of Mrs Hargreaves was highlighted earlier. She was a single parent who found that lack of services available to support her in carrying out her caring responsibilities as a parent during her periods of illness was a significant barrier to her being able to discharge her responsibilities as an active and 'competent member of society'. As she explains in this quote from earlier in the chapter, providing services designed only to meet people's personal care needs meant that there were no suitable services available for her:

> Mrs H: The nurse said to me when you go home you know, you should not go home and jump into work and that, you won't be able to, and I thought, well, who's going to do it if I don't do it? There's nobody else here to do it, you can't expect the kids to be adults, because they're not adults, they're kids. And that was the idea, that maybe they could find some way of helping me, but they couldn't. I didn't meet the criteria of their rules,

because I could make a cup of tea and I could get the dinner on, and I could get dressed myself, so I didn't qualify.

Mrs Hargreaves viewed her role as a parent as an important part of her being able to carry out her social duties: she spoke of parenting as being her responsibility. She was offered temporary foster care for her children while she was ill but felt that was not in their best interests:

> Mrs H: [The social worker] said well, you're on the list now, if you ever need us, get in contact, like for an overnight stay to look after the kids...I didn't think it would work for the kids. I didn't want to take them out of the house, anyway, there's enough upheaval in their lives as it is.

The way the provision of services centred on individuals' personal care needs and failed to take into account the complex caring relationships and duties that many disabled people had concerned Mrs Hargreaves and others. Mrs Todd and her husband provided help with personal care for each other and also supported their son, who had mental health problems. She found that the lack of available services that could support her in carrying out her caring responsibilities for her husband and son caused her some difficulties. She was particularly concerned at the lack of available help with the housework:

> Mrs T: [The nurse] said 'who have you got at home' I said my husband. 'What can he do?' I said 'He does what he can, he's had a stroke...he does what he can, he makes himself very useful and helps me as much as he can, he always has done'... [the social worker] came to see me and she said 'well what was it that you required' and I said 'someone to put the vacuum cleaner round and do heavy jobs'. She said 'sorry we don't do things like that'...I consider it wrong that you can't get people to do your vacuuming...there are people on their own with no one to do anything for them. And I think help in respect of cleaning and washing should be made available to them.

> Mr T: I mean, cleanliness in the house is obviously as important as getting the shopping done [a service that was available]. If the house goes all filthy and horrible...

Mrs Todd viewed the need to get the housework done as an

important part of the reciprocal support she offered her husband and son. Her views were shared by many people, particularly older women, who voiced the opinion that help with housework should be available to those that needed it because it was such an important part of their caring role. As Mrs Todd said:

Mrs T: Getting someone in to do the housework would be a big help all the way round for all of us. And clean the windows, something like that. I said that's all we really need, someone to vac the carpets, upstairs and down, and we'll cope with the rest. That was really all the help I wanted. I only wanted it until I began to get better.

Mrs Todd, and many other respondents, viewed carrying out housework as part of their caring duties, and spoke of them in such a way that I interpreted as being about discharging their duties as citizens. When they were unable to carry out those tasks themselves they felt that services should be available to enable them to continue with those caring tasks that they interpreted as being part of their duties as much as possible. As has been previously highlighted, Mrs Todd called this sort of help 'essential':

Mrs T: I would certainly ask why we're not allowed to have this help when it is essential. Well, I mean, if I couldn't do anything now and [husband] couldn't do anything, then I probably would approach [social services] and say well why can't I have the essential things done that I need in the house.

In an era of budget restrictions and cutbacks, housework services were among the first services to be withdrawn by both local authorities who took part in this study, as they have been nationally (Clarke et al, 1998). It is not within the scope of this book to discuss what services are and are not essential, or which should be provided by local authorities. However, it is within the scope of this book to examine how people perceived the relationship between their citizenship status and being in receipt (or not, in this case) of services. Using the citizenship framework to analyse Mrs Todd's account, it would appear that her view of the importance of being able to carry out, or have help with the 'three essentials' of cleaning, washing and shopping, sheds some light on her view of her citizenship status. If being able to carry out a task is 'essential' then it is considered to be necessary for social participation. Therefore, in Mrs Todd's framing of her duties and needs, being denied access to services which would offer her help with the housework was a barrier to her accessing her perception of a person who was discharging her social duties - a citizen. There appeared to be little space within either the assessment procedures or the delivery of services to recognise or support the role of 'citizen-the-carer' in a way that would make sense to Mrs Todd and the other respondents who shared her perception of their caring duties.

The failure of the state to support caring as a citizenship duty has been explored in more depth elsewhere (see for example Hooyman and Gonyea, 1995; McLaughlin and Glendinning, 1994) and it is linked to the gendered nature of perceptions about what constitutes an acceptable means of discharging your citizenship duties (Lister, 1997). Although there is not space to enter into the discussion here, it is clear that some people felt very strongly that caring was an important part of their citizenship duties and as such they felt the lack of services to support them in discharging those duties acted as a significant curtailment on their social participation.

Control Over the Delivery of Services and Social Participation

Even when respondents did manage to get access to services, those services did not necessarily enable them to engage in 'minimally curtailed social participation' and so did not necessarily enhance their citizenship status. Services which were arranged to suit the needs and timetables of service providers rather than service users attracted the most criticism. The most frequently cited of these was home, or domiciliary care that had been arranged through social services. People felt they had little or no control over when and how the service was provided, and that this led to feelings of frustration and dependency, rather than independence, the ability to exercise choice and control and act as a 'competent member of society'. Mr Daniels characterised the problems he had with his home carers:

> Mr D: The only thing I don't like about this type of help is that I get so many different carers and a lot of them I don't like, and a lot of them do things they aren't supposed to do. Like they come in and they talk about other clients, especially what I don't like is two women come to do my dinner (well, one woman comes to do the dinner and the other one comes to help me go to the toilet). So they both come in and they were huddled around the cooker and they were talking about other clients and what they were doing, how much work they had,

how much work they'd done, and what a pain in the butt a certain person was. And they were behaving as if I wasn't there. And that doesn't make you feel very good.

Although he was unhappy with his carers' behaviour, and despite the fact that he paid for his care through his Disability Living Allowance, Mr Daniels did not feel in control of the service he received. He did not feel treated like a citizen, a 'competent member of society', by his carers. He also did not feel able to complain about his carers' behaviour. He stated that he would prefer to be able to employ 24 hour carers himself, and thus be able to control the quality of care that he received.

Mrs Harrison was also dissatisfied with the level of care she received from her home carers:

Mrs H: I am fed up with them, I really am...I have them twice a day, morning and night, but eight out of ten of them say 'oh I haven't got time for that this morning' and that's it.

Mrs Harrison found that she had little control over variations in the quality of the care she received:

Mrs H: On Sunday I usually have a good girl and she comes around 7. She helps me have a shower. I can manage my own shower but I can't dry myself and I can't powder myself at the back, but she usually helps me do that.

However, she was told she couldn't have the Sunday carer the rest of the week because it did not fit in with the shift patterns of the home care providers. Mrs Harrison was also unhappy at the times her carers arrived:

Mrs H: The girls come to help me get ready for bed about 9 o'clock or 8.30. And then I go to bed, the cat and I...They are supposed to get my breakfast but I always get it because I have to have it within half an hour of taking my tablets for sugar... this morning the carer said she wouldn't be here until 9.30 and I was told she would be here at 9. [My neighbour] said 'do you want me to come over?' and I said yes, so she came over and she helped me to dress, which is a good job because I wouldn't have been dressed because it was 10.30 when the carer came.

Mrs Harrison found the limitations of her service provision very frustrating, particularly the limits imposed on what tasks her carers could perform. These included switching on her TENS pain relieving machine (classed as 'medical' help) and cleaning her cooker (classed as 'non-core housework'). She felt she had no input into these classifications and that they made little sense to her. The way her services were provided seemed to be designed to give her as little control as possible over them, leading her to feel that they limited rather than enhanced her social participation. She had to curtail some activities in order to fit in with the timetable of her service providers, and did not feel that her needs were being met.

Mrs Douglas found that having different home carers coming in meant it was very difficult to establish a working relationship that could meet her and her husbands' needs:

> Mrs D: You have so many different carers. I mean, this week we've got [home carer] and we've got her all the week from Monday to Friday. Saturday and Sunday I'll have somebody different. But up until now we've had different ones perhaps every day at the beginning. Now we usually have one Monday, Tuesday and Wednesday, then we have a different one Thursday and Friday, and then a different girl Saturday and Sunday. Now to me it could improve if you had 2 or even 3 girls on a rotating system. I don't say just for me, for say for one area where they get to know you and you get to know them. They know what you need, they know what you can do, they know what you want.

Not having control over the way services were provided (in this case the identity of the person providing personal care) often meant that services were insufficiently flexible to meet people's needs. Developing a relationship with a care provider that enabled the service to be delivered in a more flexible way than formal agreements with service providers could allow could formed an important element of people's ability to participate in the social world. Mrs Douglas cites an example of where this was possible in her case:

> Mrs D: For instance this morning I had to be at the doctor's at 8.30. Now, [home carer] comes in at 8.30 so I said to her, 'Don't bother this morning I won't have a shower, I've had one every day, I won't have one'. She said, 'I'll come in earlier if you want me to'. I said, 'You can come in but I will be at the doctor's'. I said, 'You can do the vegetables and you can do the

bed and you can get [husband's] breakfast, instead of getting mine, get [husband's]' which she came in and she did. And I was quite happy with that.

Developing good working relationships with service providers and being able to have control over flexible services was mentioned by many people who ended up receiving services. Mr and Mrs Rackham found that not being in control of the timetable of care provision could prove problematic when it wasn't possible for the service to be responsive to the variations in Mr Rackham's needs:

> Mr R: Sometimes I wake up and I'm not too bad, other days I wake up - we've got to do it day by day. Sometimes I wake up and I'm really rough, really ill, then virtually all the morning is taken coming round. If we go anywhere we've got to make appointments for the afternoon.
>
> Mrs R: It's perhaps because we don't set a rigid timetable. When the home carer came in, she'd come in at a certain time, she'd get him up, get him washed, get him dressed, no matter how he felt.

The lack of flexibility in the provision of the home care service meant that Mrs Rackham felt she had to provide the bulk of help for Mr Rackham herself. This had a significant impact on her social participation, as Mr Rackham explained:

> Mr R: What we've found is that my illness affects the carer in so much as the carer can't do their own thing as much as they would have done.

Some interviewees had found themselves in the position of having to provide extra care because the lack of control that disabled people had over the provision of services meant they did not meet their needs. Although only a few respondents voiced complaints about this, many of them made it clear that providing this extra help was not without some cost to their own social inclusion. Mrs Douglas found that having to provide extra help for her husband took its toll on their family life:

> Mrs D: I'd like perhaps to go, this might sound horrible, but I'd like to go and see the children, the family, just for a couple of hours break, I'm not asking for a week's holiday, I'm not

asking for a whole day, but wherever I go [my husband] comes with me because they won't let me leave him. I would like somebody to take [my husband] and do something that he would like because I can't walk far.

People were also concerned about the appropriateness of services. The problem of not being in control of the services that were received was exacerbated when those services were not culturally appropriate. Mrs Kaur, speaking through a Gujerati-speaking interpreter, explained:

Mrs K: I did tell the home carers about the shopping but the home carers are Punjabi and the type of food we need isn't what we get, so we try and do it ourselves. Because the home carers are Punjabi they are different, they are not able to understand what sort of food they should get.

One element of the appropriateness of the services available that caused concern was the quality of those services. For example, Mrs Kaur felt that the level of care her husband received from the home carers was unsatisfactory:

Mrs K: It is a waste of money giving them money to do what they do for him, because it is just a quick wash and dress him and I am quite capable of doing that myself. They only bath him twice a week.

Mrs Kaur really wanted the home carers to give her husband a proper bath, and to get access to aids such as a commode that would enable her to care for her husband properly. She felt that the service her husband received did little to increase his independence, and did not make her job of caring for him any easier. The lack of equipment and appropriate services led her and her husband to feel isolated and limited their social participation:

Mrs K: We miss being able to go out but because my husband can't walk or sit for very long in this chair it's not possible. There's no point because he'd have to come out of the car and then he can't walk.

A better wheelchair had been promised for Mr Kaur but had not been provided at the time of interview.

The timing of services was another issue raised. Delays between being assessed as needing a service and the appearance of the service had implications for respondents' social participation. One example of this was the delay in getting access to aids and equipment via the occupational therapists. The delay Mrs Douglas experienced in accessing an assessment has been discussed in chapter five. She also experienced considerable delays in receiving services and equipment:

> Mrs D: I said to [one of the home helps] you know I am still waiting for this damned toilet seat, and she said well I'll go and have a word with [social work manager]. Now that was the 13th November and I actually got it. Now, that was originally ordered for when I came home from hospital, the 22nd August.

Experiencing a delay in receiving services or equipment could be very distressing. It could mean having to have extra services (such as home carers) which were more expensive and not always designed to meet their needs. It could also have a significant impact on people's social participation. As Mrs Douglas put it:

> Mrs D: The overall problem is getting the initial help from the beginning. You want it the day you want it, you don't want it 10 days afterwards.

Mrs Douglas experienced a delay in accessing an assessment when she came out of hospital following a hip replacement operation, which meant there was a delay in accessing the services and equipment she needed to get around the house. This delay not only meant that she experienced difficulties herself (she was confined to bed with a bout of diarrhoea) which meant that her granddaughter had to provide extra help for her, but that she was unable to support her husband who therefore needed extra respite care:

> Mrs D: That is where it fell down for us. With [husband] here I look after him, but when I'm not that is when the problems start. He's on so many drugs, so many injections, blood tests and all that, diets and everything. It isn't fair to expect the children to have to do it. My daughter has always done it up to now but this time she's got a job and unfortunately she couldn't do it.

The waiting time for aids and adaptations had a significant impact on the ability of respondents to participate fully as 'competent members of society'. People reported that not only did they have to wait several months for an assessment for aids and adaptations (usually carried out by a community occupational therapist) but that subsequently the waiting time for the aids and adaptations could be anything up to a year, or longer. In some cases this meant that people had to rely on other services, such as home care services, over which they had little control. In other cases, people found that their social participation was curtailed because the lack of adaptations to their homes meant, for example, that they were unable to get out of their homes, or use the bath or toilet, without assistance. Yet when aids and adaptations did finally arrive, they could make a significant difference to disabled people's citizenship status, as discussed in the section on Practical assistance and the 'disabled citizen'. Nevertheless, with delays as long as those reported here, aids and adaptations were often effectively unavailable services, amounting to the same kind of barriers to social participation as other services that respondents perceived themselves as needing but were unable to access.

'Citizen-the-Consumer'? Paying for Services

Both local authorities had, in common with most local authorities nationally, introduced or increased service charges in the period of implementing the NHSCCA Making service users pay for the services they receive could be viewed as the introduction of consumerism into the relationship between service users and service providers. It could be argued that service charges turn a service user into a service consumer, a citizen empowered by their spending power.

However, the only people who made the link between paying service charges and being a consumer of services did so in a negative way. Those who were unhappy with the quality of the services they received did not consider that they were getting value for their money, or that the fact that they were paying for services gave them any leverage over those services. Mrs Harrison was unhappy with how much she had to pay for her services, and the lack of control she had over them:

> Mrs H: [Home help] would have been here now you see, so I said I don't want you this morning everything's been done. My neighbour over the road is very good, she's on holiday this week, so she came and helped me shower and all the rest of it, but I had to wait for her. I thought that [home help] would be here at 9 but she wasn't. I don't know where she's been but she's dreadfully slow anyway. Oh, Domiciliary Care, they charge me £98.80 every four weeks and they do nothing.

Not only did Mrs Harrison feel she was getting an unreliable service, she also did not agree with the pricing structure of the service, as she explains:

> Mrs H: They've put up my money £5.80 just because the doctor said if I got a TENS machine (I fell down the stairs nearly ten years ago, it was six weeks after my husband collapsed and died, I fell down the stairs and smashed my shoulder, I've had two operations on it but they both went wrong). So the doctor said if I got a TENS machine it would kill pain, which it does. But because they have to put that TENS machine on they charge me another £5.80 a month.

In the section on Control over the delivery of services and social participation Mrs Harrison's example was used to show how many people did not feel they had control over the quality of services. Mrs Harrison's example also shows how people did not feel they were entering into a consumerist relationship with service providers by paying for services. Not only could they not buy themselves any power over the delivery of services by paying for them, but they also did not find themselves in the position of being able to use their spending power to exercise choice over service providers, or to chose to exit the system.

They did not have any input into the way that service charges were set, either directly through democratic means, or indirectly through exercising choice as a consumer in the market. How service charges were set was a mystery, as Mrs Douglas explains:

> Mrs D: We pay for [husband] by stamps, for me we have a bill every month because mine is - how they work it out I don't know because mine is £11.60 and John's is £5.60.
>
> Q: Is that just for the one bath a week?
>
> Mrs D: Yes. But I could have a bath every day if I wanted it, for that.

People did not feel they had a voice in setting service charges. It is not within the scope of this book to examine whether citizens of the local authorities in question had a voice through the democratic process in setting service charges, but the evidence presented here does support the conclusion that paying the service charges did not give individual respondents a voice in determining the standards of care they received because, as was discussed in the previous section, they did not have any control over the services.

Nor did people, by paying service charges, necessarily buy themselves the option of exit from the relationship with service providers. Mrs Harrison explains that despite her reservations about the quality of service she received from social services, she would always go back to them:

> Mrs H: I don't know who else to go to. If you go to private people, they don't charge any more, but it's getting someone you can trust, somebody good.

The lack of a fully developed market in social care meant that people like Mrs Harrison could not use their spending power to purchase alternative services, and they were unwilling to buy services privately which had not been vetted by social services. Being able to spend your own money on services only empowers you as a consumer if you have the option of exercising choice in the market through control over services and ultimately, this means having both a choice over providers and the possibility of exiting the relationship if services are not provided to an acceptable standard. Paying service charges per se gave the respondents none of those options.

The argument that the provision of social care services is not a fully marketised relationship between provider and consumer has been developed elsewhere (LeGrand and Bartlett, 1993). Respondents agreed that the lack of choice, voice and exit from the relationship, which Barnes (1997, 1999) argues characterises the relationship between service users and providers, makes not only the social care market a quasi-market but service users quasi-consumers. Paying service charges did not turn service users into 'citizens-as-consumers'.

For some people, paying service charges appeared to act as a barrier to citizenship, because the cost of services ate into what was for many an already over-stretched budget and thus curtailed their social participation (because the money spent on service charges was not available for other things). In some cases, paying for services increased respondents' risk of poverty, which in turn increased their social isolation and marginalisation. Mr and Mrs Wilson felt they could not afford the services that they needed:

> Mrs W: I think perhaps we'd use them more if the price wasn't so high...I would have liked to have seen them within a couple of days of arriving home [from hospital] then you could

discuss what you need and what help they could give you. At a price of course...if they had come and explained [Attendance Allowance] a bit better we might have had the cash to pay for the service.

Despite wanting to be in the position of being able to afford to pay for services, the Wilsons were denied the choice of being consumers through the lack of advice on welfare benefits available to them. This is in contrast to the experience of those respondents who did receive benefits advice from practitioners, and consequently used the money to pay privately for the help they needed (for example, by employing a cleaner, or giving money to friends or family members in return for help with shopping or personal care). Mrs Harrison, for example, paid her grandson to do extra shopping for her:

Mrs H: I use the [wheel]chair quite a lot, and my grandson comes, sometimes on a Friday. Unfortunately he is out of work and he comes and he wheels me to town in the chair and we do a bit of shopping and then I get a taxi to come back. He's only a lad and he hasn't got a car so I pay him to take me to town, and then I can get the little personal things that you don't like to ask the [home carers] to bring.

Unlike the concerns she had with the formal service providers she paid for, she was more than happy with the level of service she received from her grandson. Other respondents who used their welfare benefits to pay friends or family members for providing services did not describe this in ways which would suggest the relationship was a commodified or marketised one (Baldock and Ungerson, 1991; Ungerson, 1997). Money was often seen as a way of reimbursing out-of-pocket expenses, as with Mrs Harrison and her grandson. Being able to spend their money in this way did give people a sense of citizenship and exercising choice, without it necessarily being a consumerist choice: it did not seem to be about 'buying' a service so much as about acting as a 'competent member of society' and discharging personal debts.

Being Competent to Take Risks: The Right to Refuse Services?

Being a 'competent member of society' involves exercising choice about how to participate and be included in that society (Doyal and Gough, 1991). One element of exercising choice includes making the choice to take risks and perhaps put oneself in what could be perceived (by cautious practitioners and family members) as danger. As has been discussed before, the budget restrictions that both of the local authorities in this study were under meant that services were usually only offered to people who were considered by assessors to be at risk without the services. Perhaps because of this, and because of their professional status as experts in assessing need, some practitioners found it very frustrating when people opted to exercise their choice as 'competent members of society' and refuse services.

However, people often refused services because they had a different definition of risk to that of practitioners. For example, Mr Merrick was worried about the risk of burglary with strangers coming into his home, and had cancelled his home care service:

> Mr M: One of them come here and stand here and said do you want me to cut you any sandwiches. I said no. Things have gone missing of mine. I've bought things...and I've been missing things in the home. Just before that I had a break-in and they took all my wife's wedding rings and pearls.

Other people found that they had set things up in their own home in a way that they perceived reduced their risk of harming themselves. Mrs Leith explains how she perceived her home to be a place of safety:

> Mrs L: I daren't cross the road. I don't go out alone, I'm afraid of falling over, it seems to be making me lose my balance a bit. I'm alright if somebody is at the side of me. And of course in my own home I'm alright, because I know where everything is. I can go up and down stairs, I'm very careful because I have had one or two falls.

Many blind and partially sighted respondents also pointed out the importance of having things arranged in their homes to reduce their risk of harming themselves. Accepting services which would mean physical disruption (such as moving furniture, or having to allow a stream of unidentifiable strangers into the home) could mean increasing, rather than reducing, that risk in their view. Similar problems were raised when accepting services would mean respondents having to go into unfamiliar areas (such as attending a daycare centre). Mrs Addison explains:

Mrs A: As you'll understand I've got so used to it now. But if I am in a completely unfamiliar area, you just have to look out for yourself, whether it's indoors or outdoors.

Some people felt that on balance, the risk of accepting services was greater than the risk of going without services. None of the respondents in this study were in the position of having to accept services compulsorily, as some people with mental health problems are (Rogers and Pilgrim, 1989). However, practitioners were often perceived to be in a position of authority, and could use that authority to try and persuade respondents to accept services that they were unhappy about. In chapters four and five this was referred to as the 'citizen-the-worker' approach to assessment, where respondents were considered less competent at judging their own levels of need and risk than practitioners. The example of Mr B, discussed in greater detail in chapter five highlights this:

Mr B was an older man with poor vision and mobility problems. He had asked to see the practitioner because he wanted an extra rail put in his bathroom. The practitioner examined the bathroom and said he was not happy about Mr B's safety in there. Mr B thought his safety could be improved by an extra rail but he didn't want any more help than that. He particularly did not want a home care assistant, as he would have to pay for that and he was worried about his money. The practitioner asserted that he was unhappy with Mr B's level of risk and he wanted to bring in his two sons to the assessment before proceeding. Mr B was unwilling to give the practitioner his sons' telephone numbers - he didn't want the practitioner to bother them at work and he was unhappy with the thought that they would worry about him. The practitioner refused to continue with the assessment until Mr B agreed to let the practitioner contact his sons.

In effect, Mr B was being denied the choice to take the risk of refusing to allow his sons to be involved in his assessment or the provision of services. As became clear during the assessment, Mr B was particularly concerned about the cost of services, a concern shared by many people. Many of them discussed how accepting services would entail extra costs, usually in the form of service charges, which would place great demands on their budget. Some people even felt that having to pay for services would dramatically increase their risk of poverty.

However, deciding to refuse services often had implications for the citizenship status of family and friends who then found themselves having to provide additional help. Some people described how the lack of available services curtailed their social participation (see above): this also applied when services were available but had been refused. When additional help was needed because services had been refused, people did not tend to frame their view of the 'caring' that they did as a way of discharging their duties as a 'competent member of society'. 'Caring' under such terms tended to be referred to in ways which made it clear that respondents felt their social participation had been curtailed, rather than enabling them to carry out their citizenship duties. Refusing services could therefore simultaneously be an act of a citizen making rational enforceable choices (Plant, 1992), and a way of erecting a barrier to citizenship by curtailing their opportunities for 'minimally curtailed social participation' (Doyal and Gough, 1991) for family and friends.

Competency, Services and Social Participation

This chapter has explored the way in which needs are negotiated during the assessment process between the 'community care triangle' of practitioner, carer and service user, although such delineations are sometimes unhelpful when working within a citizenship framework, as has been discussed. When viewing the assessment process through a citizenship framework, the important question is which player in the process is considered competent to assess a person's needs. Is it the practitioner as expert ('citizen-the-worker' over 'citizen-the-user'), or is it the practitioner as 'co-citizen'? The role of 'citizen-the-carer' appeared to be less important within the assessment process than was originally envisaged. However, perhaps the most interesting scenario is that which failed to emerge: that in which 'citizen-the-user' takes control of the assessment process.

The second half of this chapter was concerned with the relationship between being in receipt (or not) of services and respondents citizenship status through their ability to engage in 'minimally curtailed social participation'. The issue of control over services would appear to be vital. Where people felt they had control over services it was possible for those services to empower them and aid their social participation. However, such services had to be appropriate, of sufficient quality and be cost effective for respondents to feel this way about them. Services that were provider-driven, of variable quality and too expensive acted as significant barriers to respondents social participation and thus threatened their citizenship status.

7 Community Care Assessments in the 1990s: Citizenship Denied?

The evidence presented in chapters four to six examined the practice of assessment and discussed the experiences of disabled people and their families who attempted to negotiate access to both an assessment and services with their local authority social services department. This chapter will re-examine some of those experiences in the light of the citizenship framework outlined in chapters two and three. This encompassed three elements: the protection (or otherwise) of disabled people's civil right to an assessment (and consequently the protection or otherwise of their social rights to services); the issue of who was considered to be the most 'competent member of society' (Turner, 1993a) in the assessment process; and the issue of whether the process and outcome of the assessment resulted in disabled people and their families being able to engage in 'minimally curtailed social participation' (Doyal and Gough, 1991). This chapter will therefore address the question of whether community care policy and practice in the mid-1990s operated to protect or threaten the citizenship status of disabled people and their families.

Rationing Access

As was argued in chapter three, a community care assessment is a civil right. It is a right granted to everyone who may appear to need services under the NHSCCA. As such, it should, along with other civil rights, be enforceable using judicial mechanisms. However, unlike civil rights in other areas of welfare, particularly rights to cash benefits, the right to an assessment has never developed its own quasi-judicial process. In setting up assessment and care management as the 'cornerstone of quality community care' (Department of Health, 1989) no formal appeals procedures were put in place to give the assessment process a formalised standing. Instead, local authority social services departments were given the discretion to put in place whatever assessment and care management systems would enable them to meet their obligations under the NHSCCA.

This discretion has led to considerable variations in practices not only between the two local authorities participating in this study, but between different social services teams and even, on occasion, between different practitioners working within the same team. Although formal procedures and criteria did play a small part in determining who accessed a community care assessment, of far greater importance were the informal and discretionary decisions taken by frontline practitioners. Both the formal and informal procedures and practices were ways of ensuring that practitioners could meet their obligation to limit the numbers of people gaining access to both assessments and services, with other considerations such as user involvement and professional values having to take second place.

In chapter four these practices were analysed and broken down into three gatekeeping mechanisms: managerial (the formal criteria for who could access an assessment and services), bureaucratic (the informal processes used by some frontline practitioners to ration access to assessments as a way of rationing access to resources) and professional (the decisions made by practitioners within the assessment process about who had legitimate needs and should therefore access services). Using a typology developed by Klein and colleagues (1996) and based on that used by Parker (1975) it was shown that these various gatekeeping mechanisms are ways of rationing access to scarce welfare resources (Rummery and Glendinning, 1999). It is difficult to argue that rationing per se is a threat to any individual's citizenship status. Access to welfare goods means access to resources which are finite: the key question for any welfare state is not whether to ration access to resources but how. The issue of community care assessments, services and citizenship is not therefore that access to services is rationed, but how that rationing takes place. Specifically, do the rationing mechanisms employed by practitioners protect or threaten the citizenship status of applicants for services?

Rationing Access to Assessments

The formal criteria for accessing assessments (characterised in chapter four as managerial gatekeeping) were similar in both local authorities with one crucial difference. Local authority A explicitly recognised in its formal procedures that disabled people had the civil right to access a community care assessment. Practitioners in this authority did appear to be aware of that right, and that it was based in law. Local authority B, at the time the fieldwork took place, made no formal recognition in its procedures of the right to access an assessment. Consequently, practitioners in local authority B seemed less aware of that right, although as the evidence showed this appeared to make a difference in practice only in the Generic Team - practitioners in the teams dealing with sensory impairment appeared to operate a system whereby everyone accessed an assessment.

This failure on local authority B's part to recognise and protect disabled people's right to access an assessment was one of the more serious and obvious threats to their citizenship status. The consequences of not being able to secure access to an assessment were that disabled people had no chance of getting access to services that might increase or facilitate their social participation: in other words their access to social rights was compromised by this failure to protect their civil rights. There was no opportunity to negotiate access to services with practitioners if disabled people could not get access to the arena of negotiation in the first place.

In its operation, this failure to protect the civil right to an assessment had the most worrying consequences for older disabled people. As was seen in chapter four, practitioners in the sensory impairment teams in local authority B, and practitioners in the Older Person's Team in local authority A, behaved as though older people approaching them for assessments did not have the same civil rights as younger disabled people, even though the legislative source of the right to an assessment does not specify an upper age limit. This would suggest that an indirect ageism is in operation: the formal and informal policy and practice in social services departments is discriminating against applicants for assessments on the basis of age.

This threat to older disabled people's civil rights appears to have developed from a misunderstanding of the meaning of disabled, with managers and practitioners behaving as though that term did not apply to people over the age of 65. Yet guidance from central government following legal challenges to earlier legislation has always maintained that 'disabled' should be interpreted as widely, not as narrowly, as possible (Department of Health, 1990) and the NHSCCA made it clear that local authorities have a duty to assess the needs of anyone who appears to need their services: moreover, if a person falls within the broad definition of a 'disabled person' the local authority has a specific duty to carry out an assessment of their needs upon request (for example, see Richards, M, 1996 for further discussion of the implications of this).

Yet none of disabled people or their families were in the position to challenge either the explicit, formal managerial gatekeeping practices or the implicit, informal bureaucratic gatekeeping practices used by frontline practitioners that could prove to be a significant threat to their civil and social rights. Although formal criteria for who could access assessments was published and available to both the public and practitioners, neither party appeared to be aware of their rights or duties in this area. This may be the result of the discretion given to local authorities in setting up their assessment and care management systems, because it was in stark contrast to the level of awareness shown by both practitioners and people who received assessments as part of the formal registration process in the Blind Team.

People who had accessed assessments from the other teams which were aware of disabled people's civil rights, such as the Deaf Team and Younger Person's Team, did not share this knowledge. In these cases, people were not necessarily aware that they had been through any formal procedure that protected their civil and social rights. In contrast, people who were assessed or registered by the Blind Team were aware that they had been through a formal procedure. Arguably, this is an important element of protecting individuals' citizenship status. If people are aware that certain rights exist, and that they are going through a process that gains them access to both civil and social rights, they are in a much stronger position to ensure that their own citizenship status is protected and enhanced, rather than threatened by the process.

Similarly, the lack of awareness on the part of interviewees from the Deaf and Younger Person's Team that they had been through a formal assessment process that should have protected their civil and social rights shows that it is not necessarily sufficient for practitioners alone to be aware of, and protect, disabled people's civil right to an assessment. This becomes even more apparent when the other types of gatekeeping undertaken by practitioners are examined in more depth.

No Right to Challenge Rationing Decisions Within Judicial Process - a Threat to Civil Rights?

In practice the managerial and bureaucratic gatekeeping of the kind described above operated to exclude older disabled people from accessing assessments in the same way that younger disabled people were able to, even if many of them were not aware that this was the case. Although this arguably represented a significant threat to older disabled people's civil and social rights, practitioners, if challenged, could always assert that they had carried out a needs assessment of an applicant. This is because of the discretion given to local authorities as to what actually constitutes an assessment. Unlike the misunderstanding of the term 'disabled' (which could be easily clarified if managers and practitioners were aware of the guidance that existed) the variance in the understanding of the term 'assessment' is a direct result of deliberate central government policy. At least nine different models of assessment and care management systems were described for the benefit of local authority managers (SSI/SSWG, 1991) and as was seen in chapter four the six teams which took part in this study used a bewildering combination of systems and procedures. Because most of these procedures were informal systems developed by practitioners and managers acting as 'street level bureaucrats' (Lipsky, 1980) rather than formal institutional criteria they were referred to in chapter four as bureaucratic gatekeeping,

Practitioners and managers in the Generic and Older People's teams used a variety of bureaucratic mechanisms that were designed to limit the number of people accessing a face-to-face assessment with a practitioner. These included service-specific assessments; using risk-based criteria; and using service charges; all were ways of deflecting or deterring potential applicants for assessments. Practitioners were able to do this and still arguably fulfil their legal obligation to carry out an assessment of all applicants because no-one, least of all the applicants, could challenge them. For practitioners, the assessment began at the point of contact or referral: if they made the decision not to continue with a full face-to-face assessment following their judgement on a referral, that in itself constituted an assessment of the applicant's needs.

This type of gatekeeping is potentially a significant threat to disabled people's citizenship. It explains why so many of the respondents in this study were completely unaware that they had been through an assessment process. Although their civil rights were protected in the most basic way (in that they had accessed an assessment, of sorts) the fact that they were unaware that they had been through an assessment, or that decisions had been taken about their needs without involving them in any meaningful way, means that both their civil right (to an assessment) and their social rights (to services) had been compromised. If disabled people cannot get access to an arena of negotiating need in which they are fully aware of the meaning of the process, the fact that they have accessed an 'assessment' is of little use to them. If a 'right' to an assessment is an enforceable choice (Plant, 1992) then the fact that disabled people cannot enforce that choice means their rights are threatened.

The procedural discretion allowed to local authorities, and most significantly the lack of any systemised right to appeal community care decisions, has resulted in disabled people experiencing sometimes insurmountable barriers to citizenship, in terms of both their civil and social rights being compromised, and correspondingly their ability to participate in society being curtailed. Yet, while very few people recognised the word 'assessment' or were aware of its significance, they all shared a sense of what an assessment might be. Everyone recalled a face-to-face meeting with a practitioner, and a discussion about their needs and what services might be available to them. Those that recalled a struggle to get to this face-to-face meeting valued it highly, and were disgruntled at the seemingly unnecessary barriers that they had experienced. No-one (apart from one group, discussed below) displayed any sense of being able to challenge the barriers to accessing an assessment that they had experienced: they had very little sense that their civil rights had been infringed.

The exception to this were people who had accessed assessments from the Blind Team, whose practitioners took pains to explain to applicants that they were entering into a formal process (usually of being registered blind or partially sighted) and what that process might mean for them. As a result, these people not only were aware that they had been through a process which had implications for their citizenship status, but they felt much more able to challenge and engage with practitioners during the process of negotiating their needs. In this way, both their civil and social rights were protected by the formalisation of the registration and assessment process.

There is therefore an argument for formalising the assessment process in the same way as the registration process. This would leave front-line practitioners and managers with much less discretion to decide who should access assessments, and much less able to use bureaucratic mechanisms to gatekeep access to resources. This would serve to protect the citizenship status of disabled people (particularly older disabled people): their civil right to an assessment would be guaranteed, and they would face no significant barriers in getting to the arena of negotiating their needs with practitioners.

Practitioners in the teams which used bureaucratic gatekeeping to limit the number of people who accessed a face-to-face assessment appeared to find it a fairly stressful undertaking. They were having to make decisions about whether applicants were likely to need services on the basis of very little information. There was no room in the process for the type of reflexive negotiation about need that Cheetham (1993) thought should characterise the role of professional social workers in the assessment process. Formalising the process, and thus protecting applicants' civil rights, would also serve to ease the pressure on practitioners to act as gatekeepers to face-to-face assessments.

However, the practitioner's role as gatekeeper to scarce welfare resources would not disappear were the process to be formalised and a uniform, quasi-legal system of appeals put in place. The right to an assessment does not constitute the right to services: practitioners have a significant role to play in either protecting or threatening applicants' social rights within the negotiation of need.

No Right to Services to Meet Needs: the Conflict of Competent Informants

Unlike in the case of welfare benefits, where there is a right to a subsistence income to meet needs, within community care (or health care) there is no right to any particular services to meet needs. The professional role of workers as gatekeepers to services is an established part of the provision of welfare in Britain. As Cheetham asserts (1993) the desire for a service does not necessarily equate with a need for that service, and she maintains that the role of a professional social worker within community care should be to establish whether or not there is a need for services.

In ascertaining what constitutes a need for services, practitioners have to rely on a variety of informants, themselves included, who are considered to have a variable degree of competence in providing information on applicants' needs. The decision making process within community care assessments can have potentially life-altering consequences for applicants - it can mean the difference between being able to engage in 'minimally curtailed social participation' (Doyal and Gough, 1991) and having that social participation curtailed. In other words, the outcome of a community care assessment can mean the difference between being a citizen and a non-citizen for applicants. As such, the assessment process is one of the 'various practices' which define a person as a citizen (Turner, 1993a). It is therefore important to analyse the way in which practitioners exercise their professional judgement and discretion when making decisions about needs.

Practitioners in this study seemed to subscribe to broadly different value bases according to the type of team within which they were working. Generally, with some key exceptions, practitioners who worked within the specialist teams were working within a social model of disability, which appeared to translate into the disabled person themselves being considered one of the key competent informants on their needs. Practitioners in the specialist teams often went to great lengths to ensure that disabled people were involved in the assessment. For example, practitioners in the Deaf team would often spend a great deal of time ensuring that the method of communication used during an assessment was accessible to everyone, refusing to carry out assessments where this was not the case. This could be characterised as a 'citizen-the-user' approach to assessment - where potential service users are treated by practitioners as competent citizens, and their citizenship status protected over that of other interested parties such as carers.

On the other hand, practitioners in the hospital and generic teams were more likely to consider another professional, particularly a health professional, to be a more competent informant on a person's needs than the applicant themselves. This could be characterised as a 'citizen-the-worker' approach to assessment. Practitioners in these teams considered other workers, and themselves, to be the most competent citizens in the assessment process. However, this position was not so far removed from that of practitioners in the specialist teams. While these practitioners made a much greater effort to involve applicants in the assessment process, particularly not allowing carers to speak for disabled people, it was not the case that disabled people were considered the most competent assessors of their needs. Perhaps because all practitioners, regardless of the type of team they worked in, were always aware of their role as gatekeepers to services and resources, or perhaps because they shared Cheetham's view of their own professional role and status within the assessment process, practitioners even in the specialist teams considered themselves to be the most competent informants. Information from other sources was always filtered through their own professional judgement and discretion when making decisions about which services applicants should be able to access. All practitioners used a 'citizen-the-practitioner' approach to assessment in this way.

Practitioners in the hospital and generic teams tended to use a medical model of disability, in that they viewed the source of a disabled person's problems as being their impairment and saw their role as helping the person adjust to their impairment (Oliver, 1990). However, it is important not to generalise too much from these observations. While there appeared to be broad values subscribed to by teams (such as the model of disability) each encounter between applicants and practitioners was marked by other influences which could sometimes override the 'team' values held by practitioners. One of the most interesting influences from a citizenship perspective was that of people considered by practitioners to be carers, or potential carers. As was discussed above, practitioners in the specialist teams tended to adopt a 'citizen-the-user' approach, where disabled people's views were given greater importance than those of carers. However, they also tended to abandon this approach if it appeared to them that the disabled person was older and at risk, as was shown in the evidence presented in chapter five. When this occurred practitioners adopted what can be characterised as a 'citizen-the-carer' approach to assessing need:

considering carers to be more competent informants on need than disabled people.

While the 'citizen-the-carer' approach appeared to be a deviation from the team values in the specialist teams, for practitioners in the hospital and generic teams it was a much more commonly adopted approach. In some ways this was a pragmatic response to circumstances (for example, as a way of overcoming the difficulty many people in hospital had in making a realistic assessment of what their needs would be once they got home). However, the circumstances were often the result of practices designed to meet the needs of busy practitioners rather than the needs of applicants. For example, the practice in the Generic Team of gathering information from carers, workers and (sometimes) disabled people over the telephone seemed to be to enable practitioners to prioritise their workload rather than allow applicants the time and space to discuss their needs fully. Practitioners ended up getting most of their information from people who were in a position to give it quickly over the telephone, a practice which often favoured workers (usually fellow health or social care professionals used to communicating in this way) and more articulate applicants (usually carers, or disabled people who were long-term service users and therefore used to the system).

Even when disabled people managed to circumvent the managerial and bureaucratic gatekeeping that could threaten their civil rights, there remained significant threats to their social rights within the professional gatekeeping used by practitioners. There appeared to be a hierarchy of citizenship claims within the assessment process. Who was considered to be the more competent informant on need varied according to the values of both the individual practitioner, the 'team' values, and the status of the applicant (whether or not they were older, considered to be at risk or a carer). The most competent informant on need was always the practitioner themselves. If the role of practitioners as professional gatekeepers to services and resources remains (and there are no signs that this will change within community care policy in the UK) this is problematic for applicants for services. While they continue to have no right to any particular services to meet needs they will have to go through some kind of professional gatekeeping process, and while they have no control over either the form of the process, or the formal or informal criteria used by practitioners to decide their needs, they have no way of ensuring that their citizenship claims take priority in the hierarchy. The level of discretion that practitioners are allowed to use when carrying out their professional gatekeeping duties is therefore arguably a danger to some disabled people's social rights.

Attempting to Assert Civil Rights

In the previous section it was found that the evidence from observations of assessment practice suggested that disabled people's social rights were compromised by the type of managerial, bureaucratic and professional gatekeeping undertaken by practitioners. This section will explore what evidence the accounts of respondents in this study revealed about the impact of the assessment process on their citizenship status, particularly as they attempted to enforce their civil right to access an assessment.

The Imposition of Civil Rights?

As was seen in chapter five, some people experienced the assessment process as something that was imposed upon them, rather than something which they themselves had sought. This was particularly true of people who accessed an assessment in hospital or who were referred by someone else to social services. They did not speak about the assessment encounter in a way which made it sound as if they had accessed a civil right. In fact, many of the issues and concerns about the process raised by this group of respondents appeared to indicate that accessing an assessment in this way could be detrimental to their civil and social rights.

People who were referred to social services while they were in hospital often found themselves ill-prepared for the fleeting encounters with practitioners which constituted their assessment. Because practitioners did not usually take the time to explain the assessment process fully to patients, and did not leave their name or a way of being contacted, many people were unaware of the significance of the encounter. Can someone's civil right to an assessment be said to be protected when they are unaware that it has been carried out? It is certainly difficult to see how a meaningful dialogue about needs can take place when one party is unaware that they are participating in such a dialogue. People who had been assessed in this way complained that they had had no warning or time to prepare themselves, and were often left with unanswered questions. This group of respondents also often alluded to the fact that they felt they had unmet needs: they had wanted to access services but were not given the opportunity to articulate their needs.

This could be seen as an example of procedures being designed to meet the needs of practitioners rather than disabled people and their families in the assessment process. Within the hospital team practitioners were under a great deal of pressure to carry out a high number of assessments quickly in order to have fulfilled the local authorities' obligations under continuing care guidelines to enable people to go home from hospital and avoid blocking beds. Practitioners in the Hospital Team acted interchangeably and it would therefore make no sense to leave their name as they would not be responsible for following up any enquiries. This often left people without the necessary information to contact the team once they had had a chance to think about their needs. If we accept the point that an assessment, in order to be meaningful, had to be a recognised arena for the negotiation of need, it did therefore appear that the procedures used by the Hospital Team could, in some cases, prejudice respondents' civil right to access an assessment.

However, the procedures used by the Hospital Team did ensure that a high number of people accessed at least a basic assessment of their needs without having to wait very long. Nevertheless, the way that the assessment process was started, sometimes without the respondent being aware of it, could cause respondents concern. Some people even characterised an imposed assessment as a threat to their civil rights because it involved what they perceived to be an invasion of their privacy. Practitioners who appeared out of the blue, asking personal questions (particularly about money) and wanting to involve other family members in what some people considered to be private affairs were perceived as an unwelcome intrusion. If these practitioners then offered undesired services respondents felt that their status as competent individuals, able to decide on their own needs, was being undermined. In other words, they perceived their status as 'competent members of society' to be essentially private citizens, with minimal contact with the state, and this was compromised by the practitioner's involvement.

Yet this desire, or 'right to privacy', needs to be measured against the experiences of the group of people who experienced considerable difficulty in accessing a meaningful assessment. As was seen in chapter five this group's civil right to access an assessment was often compromised by the procedures used by practitioners. Given the vital role assessment plays in enabling people to protect their social rights and citizenship status, it is arguably preferable to impose the civil right to an assessment. This raises the question of whether civil rights which have to be imposed can be said to be rights at all. Certainly the idea of giving the state powers to enforce the right to an assessment over the right to privacy is a worrying one, as survivors of the mental health system would attest (Rogers and Pilgrim, 1989, Rogers et al, 1993). However, it is an idea considered more acceptable in some areas of the welfare state than others: the 'right' to education is one which has to be actively opted out of, for example. Given that services (and consequently service charges) could not be imposed (in the way that they might, for example, be imposed on people with mental health problems) imposing the right to an assessment does not appear to be that big a threat to civil liberties when balanced against the experiences of people whose failure to access their right to an assessment threatened their citizenship status.

However, as the experiences of people who were assessed by the Younger Person's Team and the Deaf Team shows, it is possible for the assessment to be treated as a civil right and yet not imposed: i.e. respondents who accessed assessments from practitioners in these teams had to actively seek them out but experienced no appreciable barriers in accessing an actual assessment. This would suggest that the imposition of civil rights, while it has its advantages, is not a necessary precondition for the protection of those rights.

There was a group of people whose civil rights were imposed upon them but who experienced this imposition as a positive protection of their citizenship status: those who were registered blind or partially sighted. This was a procedure set in motion by another person, usually a hospital consultant: in fact, it could not be initiated by the respondent themselves, although they could (and did) initiate community care assessments that were essentially exactly the same procedure. Yet, as the evidence in chapter five shows, this group of respondents universally welcomed the process. It was perceived as a way of opening up access to sometimes hitherto unknown social rights (benefits, equipment and services) as well as information and local networks. It was also perceived as a way of legitimating people's status as a disabled citizen: the process simultaneously legitimated people's impaired status (and relieved them of some of the duties of citizenship) whilst unlocking access to things which would help them overcome the barriers to 'minimally curtailed social participation' and thus enabled them to be full citizens, or 'competent members of society'.

The key qualitative difference between the experiences of blind and partially sighted people, and the other disabled people who had community care assessments imposed upon them, appeared to be the efforts made by practitioners to make the process as accessible and inclusive as possible. Blind and partially sighted people had all received written (or taped) notice of their assessment and practitioners took a great deal of trouble during the course of the assessment to explain what was happening and encourage respondents to discuss their needs. Practitioners also left information about how they could be contacted at the end of the assessment, and several people pointed out how important it was to be able to re-contact practitioners in this way, as they thought of new queries or their needs changed. Although their civil right to an assessment was imposed upon them, this group felt they had an ongoing relationship based on trust with their practitioner: they were treated as competent citizens.

There are other possible explanations for the apparently better practice displayed by practitioners working in the Blind Team. They were removed from the immediate stress of having to act as rationers because of the large stocks of free equipment and services to which they had access. However, practitioners in the hospital team were also not under any direct pressure to ration access to services (because they held no budget themselves for individual applicants) and they did not make the same effort to ensure that disabled people could participate fully in the process. It could be argued that the Blind Team were better trained as practitioners. However, the values that appeared to drive their practice (particularly their commitment to the social model of disability, the employment of disabled practitioners, and their commitment to ensuring that disabled people were fully included in the assessment process, sometimes to the detriment of 'carers') were shared by practitioners in other teams, particularly the specialist teams. However, while people who had accessed assessments from the other specialist teams reported some elements of good practice that would point to a co-citizenship approach to assessment (see below) it was only the blind/partially sighted people who spoke about the assessment itself in terms which I interpreted as being about accessing a civil right. It is for these reasons that I have rejected alternative analyses and maintain that the formalisation of both the imposed process of registration and the sought process of assessment was the key to the protection of disabled people's civil rights.

The powerful position of the practitioner in the assessment process means that the onus must be on them to protect the citizenship status of applicants for assessments and services, particularly when the applicant's civil right to an assessment is being imposed rather than sought by themselves. Evidence from blind and partially sighted people suggested that some practitioners did manage to achieve this despite their difficult and conflicting role within community care policy, by sharing as much information as possible and treating applicants as 'co-citizens'. However, evidence from respondents assessed in hospital and by other community teams suggested that this was not always the case and that other pressures (such as the need to clear beds, save resources or limit the number of people accessing a full assessment) took precedence over treating applicants as 'co-citizens'.

Negotiating Access to an Assessment

Chapter five explored the evidence from people who found that asserting their civil right to an assessment was often an arduous process in which they came up against barriers that they did not understand. This appeared to be the result of assessment procedures that were designed to enable practitioners and managers to meet the 'deep normative core' (Lewis and Glennerster, 1996) of community care policy (i.e. saving money) rather than making the system easy for potential service users to access. For example, the practice of gathering initial information over the telephone (which to practitioners constituted a low-level assessment, but was not recognised as accessing the arena of needs negotiation by respondents) was a way of managing the resource of the practitioner's time. However, it resulted in people who were unhappy with discussing their needs in detail over the telephone being unable to access a meaningful assessment.

Other barriers included the use of service-specific assessments (often carried out by service providers), being unable to prove they met the criteria for services (for example not being considered at risk because of the presence of someone the practitioner considered to be a carer), being made to wait long periods for an assessment, and being passed around different offices. These barriers often led to delays in accessing an assessment or being unable to access an assessment at all. Having to negotiate these barriers to their civil rights could have significant consequences for disabled people and their families, resulting in higher levels of need than was the case when they first approached social services. Yet these barriers were usually erected by managers and practitioners as a way of meeting their duty in community care policy to save money and gatekeep access to scarce resources. As was seen earlier in the discussion, no matter what approach to assessing need is adopted, practitioners will always be in the more powerful position to dictate the process than disabled people. When practitioners are not explicitly safeguarding disabled people's civil rights to an assessment, or making an effort to adopt a 'citizen-as-user' or 'co-citizen' approach to assessing needs that protects the disabled person's status as a 'competent' informant on their needs, and allow other overriding duties to take precedence, then disabled people's citizenship status will suffer.

The difficulty for many people appeared to lie in the difference in definitions between what they and practitioners would consider to be an assessment. Disabled people and their families spoke of an assessment in terms which evoked an arena of needs negotiation, usually a face to face meeting with a practitioner. They were more than happy to accept the professional gatekeeping role carried out by the practitioner, often welcoming the practitioner's expertise and ability to open up access to services, information and equipment hitherto unavailable to respondents. What was more difficult to accept was the managerial and bureaucratic gatekeeping mechanisms employed by managers and practitioners to ration access to face to face meetings with practitioners. Whilst disabled people and their families interpreted an assessment as being a face to face meeting, practitioners maintained that they started gathering information on applicants' needs from the very first contact: for them, the assessment began at the point of referral. This made little sense to people who were often unaware that they had been referred. They could not realistically participate in the assessment or negotiate their needs until they were in a situation where they had time and support to discuss their needs fully: this meant a face to face meeting with a practitioner.

However, a practitioner's time is also a resource in short supply and therefore needs to be rationed. The teams that participated in this study and did not use bureaucratic gatekeeping mechanisms had to operate a waiting list for face to face assessments: applicants on the waiting list were prioritised according to the perceived urgency of their needs so some kind of assessment did take place prior to the face to face meeting. Some people found that a delay in accessing an assessment caused them considerable difficulties and distress. The civil right to access an assessment had been upheld for them so in one sense their citizenship status was protected. However, the failure to access a timely assessment could be as problematic as failing to access a meaningful (i.e. face to face) assessment. As it was not possible for people to access services without first accessing an assessment, delays had the same effect as being denied services: people often found themselves in the position of having their ability to participate in the social world compromised because they did not have access to the kind of services, help or equipment that could enable them to overcome the physical and social barriers to their full participation in society. For some people, delays in accessing an assessment therefore threatened their citizenship status because their social rights were affected, even though, technically, their civil right to an assessment had been protected.

It would be appear from the evidence that several elements need to be in place if the process of accessing an assessment is to protect rather than threaten applicants' citizenship status. Assessments themselves must be meaningful to applicants: in other words, they must be spaces it which is it possible for applicants to negotiate and discuss their needs as fully as possible. The information-gathering process which took place prior to applicants accessing this arena cannot, therefore, be seen as constituting a meaningful assessment for applicants, even though it could and often did form the bulk of an assessment for practitioners. Accessing a meaningful assessment also meant accessing a timely assessment: delays in getting to the arena of needs negotiation were often as problematic as failing to reach the arena at all.

The Civil Right to an Assessment?

The right to an assessment is technically a civil right, granted and protected by judicial processes. In contrast, access to services is a social right, contingent upon the professional discretion of practitioners. However, the evidence in chapters five and six shows that access to a meaningful assessment is not always experienced by applicants as the granting of a civil right. Those respondents who had to negotiate access to a meaningful assessment, or found that access was barred completely because of the managerial and bureaucratic barriers they faced, experienced the process as though the assessment itself was a welfare resource that had to be rationed. Practitioners and managers appeared to be using a variety of techniques that Klein and colleagues (Klein et al, 1996) would recognise as rationing by deterrence and denial to prevent applicants from gaining access to an assessment, particularly in the generic-type teams.

It was difficult to challenge these barriers to assessment because so many of them were the result of practices that were shared by practitioners, but were nevertheless informal, implicit and not publicised, as characterised most of the bureaucratic gatekeeping mechanisms used by practitioners and managers. Even when practices were 'formal' (such as using home care managers to carry out 'home care assessments') neither the language used, nor the practice itself was explained to applicants. Informal, implicit rationing practices (such as denying applicants access to an assessment unless they asked for a specific service, or showed their willingness to pay for a service at the outset) were often effective mechanisms at deterring applicants from accessing a meaningful assessment simply because it would not have occurred to applicants to challenge the procedures. People were placed at a significant disadvantage by both their lack of knowledge of their formal, legal civil right to an assessment, and the practitioner's superior knowledge of the team's formal and informal procedures and criteria for accessing an assessment.

It appears in some cases that an assessment was treated as a rationed social right, the access to which was contingent upon the professional discretion of front-line practitioners. The erection of managerial and bureaucratic gatekeeping mechanisms appeared therefore to threaten disabled people's civil and social rights by making them fulfil additional criteria in order to access an assessment. Technically, everyone who is 'disabled' (a term which should be as interpreted as widely as possible, according to Department of Health (1993) guidance) or appears to be in need of services which the local authority provides or purchases is entitled to access an assessment. As discussed above, practitioners ensured they were operating within the letter of the law by claiming that the assessment began at the point of referral, usually long before applicants could realistically participate. In practice, having to negotiate barriers which functioned as rationing mechanisms in order to access an assessment meant that the assessment itself had become a social rather than a civil right.

The contingent nature of the right to an assessment was reinforced by the lack of a clear right to appeal the decision by practitioners not to allow applicants to access a full meaningful assessment. While all the teams who participated in this study had complaints procedures, these usually concerned applicants who had been unable to access services, rather than assessments. Moreover, this information was usually only available (if at all) to applicants who had been through the assessment process, as part of their 'care plan' documentation. Even if applicants were aware of complaints procedures, there was not usually a clear right to challenge the decision to deny applicants access to an assessment using judicial procedures, as there is using tribunals in welfare rights work within social security. While the spirit of the community care legislation may have been to treat assessments as civil rights, the practice is that they are often treated as welfare goods, access to which has to be rationed in the same way as access to any other welfare resource.

For people who attempted to access an assessment from teams who used bureaucratic and managerial gatekeeping mechanisms to ration access to assessments (the generic teams), the civil right to an assessment made no sense. Their citizenship status was therefore compromised by such gatekeeping: their civil rights were denied, and they often could not access the arena to negotiate access to services, so their social rights were also compromised. This was in contrast to the experiences of respondents who attempted to access an assessment from teams who did not use managerial and bureaucratic gatekeeping (the Hospital and specialist teams) to ration access to assessments.

People who accessed an assessment in hospital reported no problems with negotiating access to a face to face meeting with a practitioner. In fact, as discussed above, some people found that they accessed a face to face meeting when they had not necessarily wanted one, in a sense having their civil rights imposed upon them. Despite the fact that these people accessed a face to face assessment, some of them reported that this did not necessarily constitute a meaningful assessment. Because such encounters happened so quickly, with little warning, time to prepare, or time and space for respondents to discuss their needs fully, some people felt the assessment itself had not provided a proper arena for negotiating their needs. Problems such as the inability to distinguish practitioners from health professionals, difficulties in making realistic assessments of need within the hospital environment, and the lack of information on both the process and its outcomes added to the feeling of not being able to participate fully in the assessment. As such, it is questionable whether these people had accessed a meaningful assessment.

In contrast, people who had accessed an assessment from practitioners who did not use managerial and bureaucratic gatekeeping mechanisms to ration access to assessments reported how pleased they were with the quality of their encounters. They valued the time the practitioner often took to explain procedures and their meanings to them, and the way the assessment was often carried out over a number of visits or telephone calls, rather than a one-off occasion. For these people, accessing an assessment was of value in itself, regardless of whether they then accessed services or equipment. People in this group felt that their civil and social rights had been enhanced and protected by the assessment process. They had been enabled to act as 'competent members of society' throughout the assessment process and the outcome had enabled them to engage in 'minimally curtailed social participation'.

The only problem with accessing assessments raised by this group was that of the timing of assessments. Delays in accessing assessments could place people in significant hardship. However, for practitioners, delays in offering assessments to applicants whose needs did not appear to be urgent was an inevitable result of working practices. There were simply not enough practitioners with enough time to carry out full, meaningful assessments as quickly as applicants would like. The concept of a meaningful assessment therefore constituted one which was not only a face to face meeting with a practitioner, with enough time and space to negotiate needs, but a meeting which was timely and did not result in unacceptable delays in accessing urgently needed services.

Given the conflicting definitions of what constitutes an assessment, there are at least two potential conclusions to be reached about the state of disabled people's civil right to an assessment. On the one hand, if we accept disabled people's definition of a meaningful assessment it would appear from the evidence presented in this study that the civil right to an assessment has been threatened by the managerial and bureaucratic gatekeeping mechanisms employed by front-line staff. Disabled people's civil rights have been further compromised by assessment procedures designed to meet the needs of managers and practitioners to minimise costs, rather than potential service users' need to access the time and space to negotiate their needs fully.

On the other hand, if we accept practitioners' and managers' definition of an assessment (an information gathering process that begins at the point of referral) then no-one approaching a social services department is denied an assessment. Disabled people's civil rights are not compromised by the managerial and bureaucratic gatekeeping that front-line practitioners employ to enable them to meet one of their main obligations under community care, that is to control costs. Nevertheless, even if this definition of an assessment is accepted, the evidence presented in this study suggests that managerial and bureaucratic gatekeeping mechanisms have a significant impact on disabled people's social rights. As these mechanisms operate to ration access to a meaningful arena in which disabled people can negotiate their needs, being unable to get past the gates meant being unable to get access to services which would aid disabled people's social participation and enable them to overcome some of the physical, environmental and attitudinal barriers they faced.

Therefore, regardless of whether the perspective of disabled people or practitioners is adopted, the use of managerial and bureaucratic mechanisms to gatekeep access to community care assessments is of concern because it affects disabled people's citizenship status, particularly in terms of their ability to engage in 'minimally curtailed social participation'. One element that is of particular concern regarding disabled people's citizenship is the difficulty experienced by many respondents in challenging the barriers to assessment that they faced.

Implicit Barriers to Citizenship

Within the Marshallian framework of citizenship, there is no absolute right to any welfare goods or services. Resources are finite and access to welfare goods must be rationed by the appropriate welfare professional. In chapters two and three it was argued that civil rights within the welfare state were those rights which were challengeable within a judicial context, and that the right to welfare goods and services is a social right, contingent upon the discretion of welfare professionals. If this argument is accepted, then the criteria for accessing civil rights must be clear, universal and challengeable: this in itself does not mean that the existence of such criteria negates any such civil rights. For example, even in situations where access to a particular civil welfare right appears to be universal, such as health, there are always some criteria which limit, in some form, who can access that right. The 'right' to be registered with a general practitioner depends on criteria such as list sizes and catchment areas. As such criteria are designed to ensure that no one GP is forced to administer to more patients than she has the resources for, this is arguably yet another form of rationing access.

There is not necessarily an inherent contradiction between rationing access and civil rights to welfare so long as the criteria for accessing the civil right are clear, universal and challengeable. In other words, the criteria must be explicit. The evidence presented in this study suggests that many of the criteria used to decide who gains access to the civil right that constitutes a community care assessment do not fit into this category. As was discussed in chapter four only the gatekeeping mechanisms designated as managerial (such as published eligibility criteria for services) were clear and explicit. Although in practice there were variations in the way they were applied, the criteria were in theory universal and, more importantly, information about these criteria was intended to be freely available to applicants (however, it should be noted that in practice most people were not aware of them).

In contrast, the bureaucratic gatekeeping mechanisms used by frontline staff were often particular and implicit. They did not form part of any formally recognised procedures (although practitioners often behaved as though they were formal) and information about them was not intended to be available to applicants. It was often the application of bureaucratic criteria that decided whether or not an applicant gained access to a meaningful assessment. However, because such criteria were not universal or explicit it was impossible for applicants to even know about them, let alone be able to challenge them. Arguably, the use of such criteria was therefore potentially a significant threat to disabled people's civil rights. This was a concern voiced particularly by older people in this study, who were most likely to have attempted to access an assessment from teams using bureaucratic gatekeeping mechanisms. What worried people was not only that they found it so difficult to access a meaningful assessment, but that they did not understand the reasons for the difficulties they experienced. Practitioners did not share information with applicants concerning the way in which decisions were made about whether or not to offer them access to a meaningful assessment. These concerns were not necessarily shared by younger disabled people who were more likely to have attempted to access a meaningful assessment from teams who did not use bureaucratic gatekeeping mechanisms to ration access to assessments, such as the specialist teams. Within the organisational systems used by the teams participating in this study there would appear to be a form of ageism in operation: older disabled people's civil rights were under greater threat than younger disabled people's civil rights.

It should not be inferred that younger disabled people experienced unfettered access to meaningful assessments. Both groups of respondents had to negotiate access to assessments past the managerial barriers that were used by all the teams in this study. However, despite the fact that few interviewees seemed to be aware of what these were, practitioners had, when asked, shared information about these criteria and the way in which they functioned. Additional information about the managerial criteria for accessing assessments was available in written form to all applicants, although only interviewees who had been given this written information by their practitioner during the course of the assessment were aware of its existence. The salient point about the managerial gatekeeping mechanisms was that the criteria used were clear and explicit, and intended to be applied universally to all applicants. As such, it was theoretically possible to critically examine the criteria and their application using Doyle and Harding's (1992) test of 'procedural fairness'. Arguably, the threat to disabled people's citizenship status is less if this test is applied to criteria and procedures and failed (because they can be altered and improved) than if it is not possible to apply the test at all. Criteria which are implicit cannot be challenged by applicants, which increases practitioners' discretion and reduces their accountability. Therefore, the use of bureaucratic gatekeeping mechanisms is a greater threat to disabled people's citizenship status than the use of managerial gatekeeping.

Gaining Access to Social Rights: Being Competent to Assess Need

The previous section examined the way in which applicants' experiences of attempting to gain access to a meaningful assessment affected their citizenship status. This section will explore the citizenship issues which arose during the course of the assessment itself, most notably the issue of who was considered to be a competent assessor of the applicants' needs.

'Citizen-the-User' and 'Citizen-the-Worker'

Disabled people generally considered themselves to be capable of judging their own needs. They were happy to play the role of citizen-the-user in assessment encounters as they considered themselves to be competent members of society. Only a few people in this study, generally those who had been very ill in hospital at the time of the assessment, were unwilling to act as competent assessors of their own needs and wanted practitioners to carry out this task on their behalf.

Most people wanted practitioners to use their superior knowledge of the availability of services, and the criteria for accessing them, on their behalf. This lack of competency in services and procedures did not, in their view, negate their position as being competent to judge their own needs. However, many people reported that practitioners did not share their faith in their ability to judge their own needs. The power imbalance within the assessment arena meant that many people reported that practitioners were in a position to override their views and that practitioners considered themselves to be the only ones competent to judge disabled people's needs. When combined with the practitioners' superior knowledge of the procedures and criteria for accessing services, and that practitioners were in the position of deciding who should access services, in many cases it appeared that 'citizen-the-worker' took precedence over 'citizen-the-user'.

Yet this in itself is not inconsistent with a Marshallian framework of citizenship within the welfare state. Marshall always asserted that, given the finite nature of welfare resources, professionals within the welfare system would have to be responsible for undertaking some form of rationing or gatekeeping of resources. In chapter four this was characterised as professional gatekeeping, as distinct from the managerial and bureaucratic gatekeeping discussed above. Practitioners, as welfare professionals, will always be in a position to know more about the criteria for and the availability of services than applicants. This element of the practitioner's role appeared to be acceptable: what was less acceptable was the way in which some practitioners extended this role to place themselves in the position of being more competent to judge applicants' needs than applicants themselves. The second element of citizenship, that of people being considered to be 'competent members of society' (Turner, 1993a), is important here.

The extension of the practitioners' acknowledged expertise in services into the area of assessing need is consistent with the social work profession's view of their role within community care assessments (Cheetham, 1993; Sheppard, 1995). Cheetham asserts that a desire for a service on the part of an applicant does not necessarily equate to a need for that service, and that applicants need the assistance of trained professionals to uncover their real needs. Cheetham would therefore appear to endorse the position of 'citizen-the-worker' taking precedence over 'citizen-the-user' in the assessment process. The evidence from this study suggests that there is not universal acceptance amongst disabled people and their families of this view of the practitioner's role.

Where there was conflict between practitioners and interviewees over the latters' needs it was clear that disabled people and their families questioned the idea that the practitioner was in a better position to judge the their needs than the disabled person themselves. This position only made sense if needs were equivalent to services: in other words, if a service-led assessment, rather than a needs-led assessment were being carried out. In that case, the practitioner's superior knowledge of services, procedures and criteria meant that the 'citizen-the-worker' approach assessment was a rational response. However, service-led assessments are contrary to Department of Health guidance, and to respondents' views of the nature of meaningful assessments (and to Cheetham and Sheppard's view that the role of professional social workers within community care must be more than just matching applicants with resources). A 'co-citizen' approach (see below) to assessing need appeared to be much more acceptable to respondents, and more in keeping with a needs-led assessment, than the 'citizen-the-worker' approach to assessing applicants' needs.

The Community Care Triangle?

Biggs (1994) has argued that an individualistic approach to citizenship has led to what he calls a tripartite approach in assessment situations. Because an individualist notion of citizenship does not allow for people to receive help and support without being construed as being dependent, he maintains that three possible scenarios develop: either the life-task collusion scenario (where the worker and carer collude against the user); family solidarity (where the user and carer collude against the worker); or the heroic defence scenario (where the user and worker collude against the carer). Depending on such elements as the age of the applicant and the type of team the practitioner was working in, on occasion practitioners in this study would adopt a 'citizen-the-carer' approach (what Biggs would call the life-task collusion scenario) where carers were held to be more competent assessors of need than the applicants themselves. Even in situations where practitioners would normally adopt a 'citizen-the-user' approach to assessment (such as those working in the specialist teams), the 'citizen-the-carer' approach could take precedence where practitioners considered the applicant to be at risk.

If we follow Morris' argument that the community care reforms were designed to institutionalise and support family care, and as such were incompatible with the notion of empowering users of services (Morris, 1997), then the adoption of the 'citizen-the-carer' approach to assessment is perfectly rational. It is a useful way for practitioners to meet their obligations to reduce expenditure and support family caring under community care. However, despite the fact that practitioners in this study often used this approach, it did not make any sense to disabled people. No-one reported, even when specifically prompted, that practitioners had colluded in any way with their carers against them in establishing what their needs were.

In part this may be because Biggs' scenarios do not allow for the complexities of people's relationships. His delineation of applicants into users and carers was too simplistic: interviewees in this study reported that they themselves often did not recognise, or think or themselves in such terms. Instead, they experienced a range of relationships with the family members and friends who would be designated as 'carers' by practitioners. Usually these relationships involved an element of reciprocity: many 'users' considered themselves to have caring responsibilities and many 'carers' were themselves frail or impaired and in need of support. This echoes observations made by Lister (1997) and Finch (1989) that the state can encounter problems in implementing social policies based on morally derived normative assumptions about what constitutes acceptable behaviour within family life when citizens do not share those normative assumptions. Particularly in the case of spouses it would be more accurate to say that interviewees saw themselves as a family unit, with the practitioner as the outsider (a sort of 'citizen-the-family' approach?). The picture which emerged from interviewee's accounts was not of a community care triangle, with three players vying for competent-citizenship status, but a bi-partite scenario, with the family attempting to negotiate access to services with the practitioner.

The problems encountered by respondents when they attempted to negotiate a system which could not account for the complex and reciprocal caring relationships which they experienced were documented in chapters five and six. It could lead to delays in accessing assessments (and therefore in accessing services) while different branches of social services argued about whose responsibility it was to provide the assessment, with the result that people's social participation was threatened. It could also mean that services, even if they were available, were unsuitable because they were not designed to be used by disabled people who also had caring responsibilities.

The Practitioner as 'Co-Citizen'

Both the 'citizen-the-user' and 'citizen-the-carer/family' scenarios discussed above work on the assumption that there is an inherent conflict within the assessment process between the practitioner and the person attempting to negotiate access to resources. However, some of the respondents in this study pointed out that the assessment arena did not necessarily have to be a location of conflict over who was considered to be the most 'competent member of society' to judge an applicants' needs. A partnership-based approach to assessment was more acceptable to people than one based on an assumption of conflict.

Most interviewees in this study accepted that the practitioner's knowledge of the availability of services, aids and support was superior to their own. They often expressed gratitude that this was the case, pointing out that the practitioner's alleviation of their lack of knowledge in this area was the most beneficial aspect of the assessment process. When practitioners shared this information openly it felt to people as though they were being treated as 'co-citizens'. They were treated as though they were the experts on their own impairment and needs, and practitioners were the experts on services, aids and adaptations to help overcome the barriers to social participation that were experienced by applicants. Both parties in the assessment arena had different, and equally respected, areas of competency and there was therefore no need for the assessment to be an arena of conflict, or for a 'hierarchy' of claims to citizenship.

Whilst practitioners in these 'co-citizenship' approaches to assessment shared a superior knowledge of criteria and procedures with practitioners using 'citizen-the-worker' scenarios, they did not use this superior knowledge as a way of erecting barriers and rationing access to their time and services. In fact, within a 'co-citizen' approach, criteria and procedures seemed to assume a much lesser importance overall. Where they were relevant (for example where respondents expressed a desire for a service that they did not meet the criteria for, or procedures meant that there was a delay in accessing a service) this was usually explained and for the most part the explanations were accepted in the spirit of partnership and information sharing that characterised the 'co-citizen' approach.

The 'co-citizen' approach to assessment did appear to be more commonly used by practitioners within the specialist-type teams, although a causal link between team type and the 'co-citizen' approach to assessment should not necessarily be inferred. It did appear to be used occasionally by practitioners working in other team types, and it was not unknown for practitioners in the specialist-type teams to adopt a 'citizen-the-worker' approach (see example 11 in chapter four). However a 'co-citizen' approach took a lot of time, dedication and effort on the part of the practitioner to establish, and it did appear to be a difficult approach to adopt when there was pressure to carry out assessments as quickly as possible, or to limit applicants' access to assessments as a way of limiting resource expenditure. The 'co-citizen' approach to assessment seemed to rely on an element of trust being built up between applicants and practitioners. It would appear that where applicants were considered to be potential drains upon resources that practitioners have the responsibility for, there was less incentive for practitioners to put in the time and effort it took to make a 'co-citizen' approach to assessment work.

Although a causal link between team-type and the adoption of a 'co-citizen' approach cannot be inferred, there did appear to be some elements of management practice that supported practitioners to adopt it. Practitioners who worked in teams that used a social model of disability, that had access to a wide range of resources (including aids, equipment, services, networks, benefit checks, voluntary agencies), who were not under direct pressure to ration access to resources, who were themselves disabled or worked alongside disabled practitioners (which led to better empathy between practitioners and disabled people), all appeared to be more likely to adopt the approach than others.

The 'co-citizen' approach to assessment does retain a role for the practitioner as a well-trained welfare professional. However, it is not necessarily the social work role that both Cheetham, Sheppard and other commentators have envisaged for professionals within community care. The expertise assigned to the practitioner using a co-citizenship approach is not their superior ability to distinguish a desire for a service from a need (Cheetham, 1993) or to enable applicants to 'discover' their needs (Sheppard, 1995). The practitioner's expertise lies in their superior knowledge of the services, aids and adaptations, and the criteria and procedures necessary to access them, that will meet the needs presented to them by applicants. In other words, a practitioner who worked successfully as a 'co-citizen' within the assessment process would be more of a service broker than the traditional professional social worker envisaged by Cheetham and Sheppard. Whilst such a role would encompass many of the traditional values associated with social work (such as advocacy and anti-discriminatory practice), many interviewees felt that the key element of a successful co-citizenship approach was that practitioners did not set themselves the task of being the expert in defining applicants' needs, but shared their expertise in identifying services to meet those needs. This could be done more easily if practitioners had access to a wide range of service on behalf of applicants and if the direct pressure to ration access to resources was removed.

Services and Social Participation

This final section will critically examine the relationship between the outcome of the assessment process and the citizenship status of disabled people and their families. The particular issues highlighted in chapter six included: the role the assessment played in granting applicants the status of a disabled citizen; caring; control over appropriate services; and consumerism in community care.

The Disabled Citizen

Some people in this study had been trying to cope with a worsening impairment for some time prior to the assessment process. In chapter six some of them described the barriers to social participation that they faced on a daily basis. These ranged from the social and attitudinal (such as people's attitudes to their impairment) to the environmental and physical (such as inaccessible homes and shops). Some people reported that the outcome of the assessment process had a positive impact on their perception of their own status as a disabled citizen in two important ways.

Firstly, those people who had been through a formalised assessment process (particularly those who were 'registered' blind or partially sighted) reported that this process served to legitimise their impairment. These respondents found that they no longer had to try and hide or make excuses for their inability to do some things in the way they used to. This legitimisation of their impaired status was reported positively by people who felt it freed them from some of the duties associated with citizenship that they now found difficult to fulfil, such as the duty to park in spaces not set aside for disabled people. However, perhaps more importantly, the legitimisation of their impairment also led to a reduction in the social isolation that many people reported they had experienced prior to the assessment process. They discovered that they had something in common with other people who shared their impairment: they gained access to membership of a community that was often previously unknown to them. Many of them found that participation in this new community compensated in part for the diminished participation they felt they enjoyed in their old community. People who reported this type of outcome particularly valued it when their practitioner was also part of this new community: it added to the sense that the practitioner was a 'co-citizen'.

People also valued it when practitioners, in their role as 'co-citizens', took the time and patience throughout the assessment process to explain the way a social model of disability could be applied to their particular situation. Biggs' assertion that individualised notions of citizenship lead to unwelcome dependency upon others (Biggs, 1994) explains why some people felt that the barriers to social participation which they faced in society were the fault of themselves and the result of their impairment. When practitioners persuaded them that this was not the case, and that the barriers they were experiencing were external and socially constructed (Oliver, 1990), they reported a feeling of relief. They were left with a sense that their status legitimated their need for assistance, rather than with a sense that their need for assistance meant they were dependent and not fulfilling their duties as citizens.

Secondly, some people reported that the status of a disabled citizen afforded them by the assessment process unlocked access to a range of aids, adaptations, benefits and services which enabled them to overcome some of the barriers to social participation that they faced. However, this link between acquiring the status of a disabled citizen and thus gaining access to services which aid social participation relies on the assessment process granting applicants that status. It would appear that this link only operates when the assessment process is clear, explicit and formalised. People who did not experience the assessment process in this way did not report the acquisition of the status of a disabled citizen and its associated benefits.

It should be noted that community care assessments as presently constructed are not intended to convey the status of disabled citizenship upon applicants. Community care assessments are not linked to the system of disability registration which has been declining in popularity since its inception and is now largely defunct. Within the remit of this study, theoretically only people being registered blind or partially sighted by the Blind Team experienced the formal link between their status and the assessment process. However, not everyone who accessed an assessment from this team was being registered, and the link between status and the assessment was also noted by respondents who had accessed assessments from other teams. The key appeared to be a combination of formalisation of process coupled with a practitioner as 'co-citizen' approach to assessment.

The Caring Citizen

At the time the fieldwork for the study was being carried out the 1995 Carer's (Services and Recognition) Act, giving carers the same right to access an assessment as disabled people, had not been implemented so it was not possible to assess the relationship between assessment procedures and carers civil rights. Nevertheless, the sixteen respondents in this study who would be designated by practitioners as carers (whether or not they would chose such a term to describe themselves) presented evidence which suggested that assessment procedures were not designed to cope with carers' needs. Systems of resource allocation for services could not allow for the fact that many disabled people had caring responsibilities. For most people in this situation there were no suitable services that would support them in their caring role.

As has been discussed above, the formalisation of procedures coupled with the adoption of a practitioner as 'co-citizen' approach to assessment could effectively protect disabled people's citizenship status despite the conflicting pressures within the assessment process. However, there did not appear to be an equivalent way of protecting the citizenship status of carers. Applicants had to be either 'users' or 'carers' within all the assessment procedures in this study: there was no space to allow for the complex reciprocal caring arrangements that were a feature of the lives of many people. Services (and the funding for services) were, for the most part, designed for individual service users and could not be adapted to meet the needs of carers, particularly if the carers were themselves disabled.

For some people the most significant threat to their citizenship status was the fact that the assessment process did not allow for the way in which many carers viewed the provision of help as being part of their citizenship duties. These respondents described their caring duties in ways which made it clear that they considered them to be an important part of their social participation. They did not necessarily want to gain access to services which would replace the caring tasks that they carried out, but they did want to gain access to services which would enable them to continue carrying out those tasks. Such help was often considered, in the words of one respondent, 'essential'. However, these respondents found that in many cases such services did not exist, or were designed in such a way as to be inappropriate for carers.

The problems of lack of suitable services leading to diminished social participation was no less acute for carers than it was for disabled people. In fact, those respondents in this study who were disabled and had caring responsibilities found that the inability of practitioners and assessment systems to allow for their situation resulted in a double threat to their citizenship status. Not only did they suffer diminished social participation as a result of the lack of suitable services to meet their own needs, but they also were hindered in carrying out their caring-citizenship duties by the lack of suitable services to support them in this role. They experienced barriers to citizenship both as a disabled person and as a result of isolation that was caused by having to carry out caring duties with insufficient support.

Control Over Appropriate Services

When people had succeeded in negotiating access to services one of their main concerns was the level of control they had over those services.

Services tended to be organised to meet the needs of providers, rather than users, which left people feeling as though they had little control over the quality of the service they received. Issues such as the identity of home carers, the range of tasks it was possible for them to carry out and other aspects of service delivery were decided by practitioners and service providers. Many people reported that this resulted in them having to limit or alter some elements of their social participation in order to fit in with the pattern of their service delivery. There was particular concern about the lack of flexibility in service provision.

The timing of service delivery, both in terms of how long applicants had to wait before the service started and what times it was delivered when it did start, was often reported as a crucial element of whether or not services enabled respondents to engage in 'minimally curtailed social participation'. Services that arrived too late were often perceived as being as bad as not receiving a service at all: both situations were reported to lead to people experiencing additional hardship and barriers to social participation and, in some cases, having to pay for additional services while they were waiting for an aid or adaptation to arrive. Many people were also concerned about the cost of services which could increase their risk of poverty, further curtailing their opportunities for social participation.

Therefore, respondents' citizenship status could be threatened rather than enhanced by the delivery of inappropriate services the delivery of which they had little or no control over. However, some people reported that they were experiencing the opposite scenario. Where services, aids and adaptations provided people with valuable practical assistance, were available in a timely and cost-effective manner and, most importantly, under the control of applicants, they reported that such services significantly enhanced their social participation. Often people found themselves gaining a renewed sense of independence as a result of the provision of such services. They found ways to overcome some of the physical and social barriers that had been impeding their full citizenship and social participation.

In the parlance of community care rather than citizenship, applicants found that their independence was increased by services which were needs-led rather than provider-led. It is a measure of the gap between rhetoric and reality in community care that not only did only a minority of interviewees report that their services fitted this mould, but also that a significant number of such services, aids and adaptations were provided by the specialist-type teams (and in the case of services, aids and adaptations accessed through the Blind Team, the voluntary rather than state sector) whose modus operandi often differed radically from their colleagues in other social services departments. It would appear that needs-led assessments and services were the exception rather than the norm within mainstream social services.

Evidence from the experiences of users of direct payments in the UK (where disabled people receive cash rather than services from local authorities, and then buy and manage their own services, usually through employing a personal assistant) suggests that this group of disabled people also experience enhanced choice and control over their services, and thus enhanced citizenship status (Glendinning et al, 2000; Zarb and Naidash, 1994). Being able to pay for services themselves seemed to buy direct payments users the ability to control the quality (in terms of appropriateness, timing and identity of provider) of the service, which would appear to be instrumental in whether services were a barrier or support to disabled people's citizenship status.

'Citizen-the-Consumer' in Community Care

Some aspects of the implementation of the community care changes appeared to be intended to marketise the provision of community care to make it more effective at meeting the needs of service users. The introduction and extension of service charges was potentially such an aspect: through paying for services, service users could be transformed into community care customers, being empowered through their spending power. As such, consumers within community care would be able to affect the provision of services through operating in a quasi-market and exerting choice. As making choices is a crucial part of social participation, arguably such consumers would gain an enhanced citizenship status compared to simply being service users.

The issue of service charges was a worrying one for interviewees, many of whom were on low incomes and concerned about the impact paying such charges had on their limited budget. Having to find the extra money for service charges increased some people's risk of poverty, and thus increased their risk of social isolation. Having to pay for services per se was therefore often a curtailment to their social participation and thus a risk to their citizenship status.

However, the evidence in this study suggests that paying service charges was an unsuccessful means of introducing empowerment through consumerism to respondents. As was discussed above, in order to enhance their citizenship status by enabling them to engage in 'minimally curtailed social participation', services had to be appropriate in terms of quality, timing and cost, and most importantly, be under the control of respondents. Paying for services (in the guise of service charges) in itself it did not give respondents the ability to exert control over them. The lack of a fully developed market in service providers meant that respondents were unable to exercise realistic choices and exert their spending power through the ability to exit the system and shop around for the most competitive provider. Any exercise of choice over service providers was usually carried out by the practitioner or manager on the respondents' behalf.

Respondents were also unable to exert any control over the quality of the services they received. Decisions about who should provide services, and what they were able to provide, were made by service providers and practitioners rather than disabled people. Disabled people and their families also had no input into (and very little understanding about) either the level of charges set, or the way contracts for service providers were set up. Paying for services did not appear to grant them any voice in the system.

The evidence presented in this study shows that paying service charges did not turn service users into consumers as it did not grant them the elements of choice, exit and voice necessary for a consumerist relationship to work. This supports the misgivings Barnes (1997; 1999) and others have voiced about the policy of introducing privatised and marketised systems into the welfare state. She argued that service users within such a system are at best quasi-consumers enjoying none of the advantages that should be experienced by an empowered 'citizen-the-consumer' exercising choices in a consumerist way through their spending power.

However, the experience of direct payments users again that shows being in control of money gives disabled people the power to purchase control over services, and therefore enables them ensure that services are appropriate, timely and of sufficient quality (Glendinning et al, 2000a; Morris, 1997). Although there are concerns about the low takeup, underfunding and lack of support that direct payments users experience, evidence suggests that they are more able to construct flexible, adaptative packages of care that enhance their social participation than the users of traditional statutory services, particularly in areas such as caring, leisure activities and health-related services (Glendinning et al, 2000). Whilst it is right to be cautious about the limitations of a marketised approach in empowering welfare users, it does appear that some elements of consumerism do enable disabled people to enjoy greater social participation, and therefore enhanced citizenship status.

Citizenship Denied?

The evidence suggests that at their best, assessment systems can protect and enhance the citizenship status of applicants. There are ways in which the Marshallian notion of the relationship between civil and social rights can be protected by community care assessments. The key to this success appears to lie in having clear, explicit and challengeable criteria and procedures, which would facilitate the protection of disabled people's civil right to an assessment. The evidence in this book also suggests that there is the possibility of protecting the social rights of disabled people and their families within community care assessments. This is primarily by practitioners adopting a 'co-citizenship' approach to assessment, where their expert knowledge of both procedures and the availability of services is matched by disabled people's expertise on their own needs, and thus there is no conflict within the assessment system over who is considered to be the most 'competent member of society'. The citizenship status of disabled people and their families, in terms of them being enabled to engage in 'minimally curtailed social participation' was enhanced by the provision of aids, adaptations and services that were flexible, appropriate and under the control of applicants. However, the evidence also suggests that this citizenship-enhancing combination does not appear to be universally available to applicants entering the assessment system. Some people experienced procedures and criteria which were particular, implicit and non-challengeable; practitioners constructed a conflicting hierarchy of claims to competent citizenship status within the assessment, usually with themselves as the most competent (adopting a 'citizen-the-worker' approach); and services, if accessed, were often inappropriate in terms of quality, timing and cost and were therefore experienced as a threat to respondents social participation because of the lack of control disabled people and their families could exert over them.

The next chapter will examine the policy options for community care assessments in the light of this evidence. Is it possible for the citizenship status of applicants to be protected and enhanced by community care assessments within the British welfare state as it is presently constructed? What does the evidence presented in this book about the way in which disabled people and their families experienced access community care assessments tell us about the wider relationship between disabled citizens and the state within the context of current community care policy?

8 Assessment and Care Management Policy and Practice in the New Millennium: Towards a New Framework of Citizenship?

In this final chapter, I will now discuss the policy and practice options indicated by the findings discussed in the previous chapters within the context of community care policy as part of the current British welfare state. Although the evidence presented in this book is only relevant to English community care policy and practice, the issues and concerns highlighted by the practitioners, disabled people and their families who participated in this study raise questions about community care policy as a whole. These issues fall into four main areas: the protection of the civil right to an assessment; the nature of the assessment process; the training implications for assessors; and the role of services in enabling disabled people and their families to engage in minimally curtailed social participation.

The Civil Right to an Assessment

The Problem of Variable Access to Assessments

Some people in this study found it significantly more difficult than others to access a community care assessment. There are several reasons why this variable access to an assessment has developed. Firstly, where there was not explicit acknowledgement of disabled people's right to access an assessment in the formal criteria (or managerial gatekeeping) practitioners appeared either unaware of the right, or unwilling to enforce it on disabled people's behalf. Secondly, even where practitioners were aware of the right many of them usually (mistakenly) thought it did not apply to older disabled people in the same way as younger disabled people. Thirdly, an issue that will be discussed more fully in the next section, what actually constituted an assessment (and therefore what constituted accessing an assessment) was decided by local authority managers and to a lesser extent practitioners, not by disabled people or their families.

These variations can all be explained by the degree of discretion in designing and implementing assessment systems that has been left to local authorities under community care policy. This discretion was in part intended to maintain the autonomy of local authorities and to enable to respond flexibly to levels of local need (Blackman, 1999). However, it was also intended to enable local authorities to comply with the 'deep normative core' of the policy to curb expenditure on social care services (Lewis and Glennerster, 1996) by being able to refine and alter their systems in order to balance the number of people accessing assessments and services and the quantity of services the local authority could afford to provide. Assessment systems designed to meet this aim could not also meet the aim of empowering potential service users (Ellis, 1993). In many cases the use of bureaucratic gatekeeping mechanisms to prevent disabled people from accessing a community care assessment presented a fairly significant threat to their citizenship status, both by denying their civil rights (to access an assessment of their needs) and, correspondingly denying them social rights (the ability to access services to meet their needs). This has particularly worrying consequences for older disabled people: the fact that bureaucratic gatekeeping appeared within the context of this study to be used more often in generic/older person's teams than in those specialist teams focusing on younger disabled people means that the discretion given to local authorities had the effect of introducing indirect ageism in assessment systems and community care practice.

Bureaucratic gatekeeping mechanisms, by rationing access to assessments rather than services, also proved problematic for practitioners. They meant that a great deal of practitioners' time and energy were expended on the task of deflecting demand for services and resources by dissuading applicants from pushing for a full assessment of their needs. This does not sit easily with Cheetham (1993) or Sheppard's (1995) view of trained social workers within the context of assessment and care management uncovering need as a reflexive process. Ellis (1993) also found that practitioners found it difficult to 'square the circle' of professional practice, user empowerment and rationing access to resources within the assessment process.

If disabled people's social rights to services to meet their needs and enable them to engage in minimally curtailed social participation is to be protected, a vital first step is to protect the civil right to an assessment of those needs. Although a great deal of the current focus on 'social exclusion' is on exclusion from the job market as a way of tackling poverty, arguably the issue of disabled people's exclusion from society because of the failure of the state to enable them to access the services and support they need to enable them to engage in minimally curtailed social participation demands similar attention (Rummery, 2000).

Welfare Rights and Assessments

One approach that could be used to tackle the effect of bureaucratic gatekeeping in rationing access to assessments would be to treat community care practice in the same way as social security practice, and develop a strong welfare rights ethos within community care. Welfare rights work concentrates on illuminating the complex social security system to enable people, particularly those living in or at risk of poverty, to claim social rights against the state, by reducing the power inequalities inherent in a system reliant on welfare professionals to administrate it because of its bureaucratic complexity. Many local authorities see welfare rights work as entirely consistent with user empowerment and anti-poverty strategies and thus sometimes fund welfare rights workers themselves. Claimants are assisted in making claims for social security benefits against the state, and discretionary decisions made by welfare professionals are challenged within a quasi-judicial system (such as appeals tribunals). However it should be noted that social security budgets are both demand-led and not the responsibility of local authorities, in contrast to the explicitly cash-limited budget for social care managed by them, and thus welfare rights would not be able to operate in exactly the same way with social care as with social security benefits.

Nevertheless, the right to access a community care assessment (as distinct from social social care services) is a civil right it should, theoretically, be challengeable and upholdable within a judicial context. There should be scope to extend the practice of welfare rights work to encompass community care assessments and offer support and protection to disabled people in the same way as to social security claimants. However, in practice there are several key obstacles and limitations to adopting a welfare rights ethos in community care.

The first obstacle is that despite the fact that the right to a community care assessment is enshrined in and protected by law, neither local authorities nor disabled people themselves seem to be particularly aware of that fact, nor of the rights and responsibilities incumbent on the parties concerned. This study showed that whether or not disabled people had their civil right to an assessment protected depended much more in the implicit, bureaucratic mechanisms employed by teams and individual practitioners to manage demand for resources than on the explicit managerial gatekeeping enshrined in eligibility criteria. Welfare rights can only work within the context of explicit and universal criteria that are applied with some degree of objectivity. Where it can challenge the discretionary decision making undertaken by welfare professionals it does so by holding such professionals to account by placing the onus on them to show that the relevant decision was made fairly using the appropriate criteria (within the law this principle is known as judicial review). In other words, welfare rights could only ever challenge decisions made on the basis of formal, explicit managerially defined criteria and gatekeeping mechanisms. However, that accounts for only a small proportion of the relevant decisions made about who should access a full community care assessment.

The second key barrier to extending welfare rights work to cover community care assessments is closely related to the first. It hinges on the discretion and therefore considerable variation left to local authorities in designing their assessment and care management systems. What constitutes a full assessment therefore varies not only from local authority to local authority, but between individual teams and practitioners within that authority. An assessment is not therefore a universally recognizable welfare good in the same way as, say, a sum of money or even a specified service.

In some respects it is important not to forget that this can have advantages for both managers, practitioners and disabled people and their families. If there were one prescribed type of assessment there would be little opportunity for managers and practitioners to develop the kind of responsive good practice that was valued by disabled people precisely because it was flexible and allowed them the time and space to articulate and discover their needs with the practitioner's help. A uniformly proscribed assessment system might look like the quick and faceless one operated by the hospital team, where practitioners acted interchangeably and disabled people had little opportunity to prepare themselves or fully participate in articulating and discovering their needs. It might also look like the formulaic telephone assessment objected to by applicants to the generic/older person's team, which could have been undertaken by anyone with a list of the appropriate service-driven prompts.

A third potential barrier is that welfare rights work, even when funded by local authorities, is helpful in supporting claimants against an outside party (in the case of benefits advice, the Department of Social Security). There are obviously some problems in applying such a model to community care, where the responsibility for providing access to assessments and services lies within the local authority. For welfare rights workers to be able to act as true advocates for disabled people within community care they would have to be able to operate at some arm's length from local authorities, or be completely independent of them.

The variation in what was considered to be a full assessment between teams and local authorities, and more importantly the dissonance between what was considered by practitioners and disabled people and their families to constitute a full assessment is a concern because, as this study shows, it can have a considerable impact on disabled people's citizenship status. The potential to develop welfare rights as a mechanism to protect disabled people's citizenship in the assessment process would be improved if certain key aspects of that process were changed.

The Nature of the Assessment Process

It has been argued that the variation in assessment forms and procedures used nationally is one reason why there are considerable differences in the range and type of people who are able to access a full assessment of their needs and, correspondingly, variations in the range and type of services received (Audit Commission, 1996). This study has shown that there is no one recognizable welfare good that can be defined as an 'assessment', which caused disabled people and their families concern, and was in itself a barrier preventing them from accessing their civil and social rights.

What Should Assessments Look Like?

Managers, practitioners and disabled people and their families all had very different ideas about what constituted a full assessment. For practitioners the assessment, no matter what the formal procedures were, tended to begin at the point of referral. This meant that assessments could begin and end without the disabled person themselves being involved in any significant way or even registering that an assessment had taken place. This was particularly the case in teams that used procedures such as telephone assessments or service-specific assessments.

Clearly, in order for an assessment to be meaningful to all parties, they must at least be aware that it has taken place. Given the crucial role the assessment plays in accessing services and equipment to meet disabled people's needs and therefore the role it plays in enabling them to participate as a competent member of society, it is important that disabled people can participate fully in an assessment that is meaningful to them. Moreover, practitioners who used mechanisms that mitigated against such participation, such as telephone or service-specific assessments, were also likely to adopt a 'citizen-the-worker' approach to assessing need (see below). This would appear to be entirely rational and consistent with such an approach, because if the practitioner is the person 'most competent' to assess the disabled person's needs, the full involvement of the disabled person themselves becomes less important.

However, if we are to conceptualise the assessment as the arena of negotiating needs, a conception recognised by most of the interviewees and some of the practitioners in this study, then the use of mechanisms which mitigate against disabled people's full participation in the process should be avoided. Most of the disabled people and their families in this study viewed an assessment as a face to face meeting with a practitioner - or , even better, with a range of practitioners from the different agencies responsible for providing services. It was only during face to face meetings that respondents felt able to properly enter the arena of negotiating need, because they were given the time and space to articulate their needs and explore the options properly, rather than having to decide in a brief period whether or not they wanted one specific service.

Many of the disabled people in this study were clear about what constituted a 'proper' assessment. Just as important as the face to face and sufficient time elements discussed above was the issue of information. People wanted to come away from assessments with sufficient information to enable them not only to make choices between service or equipment options, or choices about whether to accept services or equipment, but also information about the process of the assessment: how to contact the practitioner again, what to do if circumstances changed, what was happening to their application and how long the process might take. They therefore wanted to be significantly involved and kept informed about both the process and the outcome of the assessment. Particularly, they wanted to understand the basis upon which decisions about their needs and the availability of, and their suitability for, services and equipment were made. If they received or were refused a particular service or piece of equipment they wanted to know why, and they wanted to be able to challenge that decision if they thought it was unfair or did not accord with their own perception of their needs.

In other words, disabled people and their families wanted the assessment process to be fair and explicit. The group of respondents who expressed the greatest satisfaction with the assessment process (as distinct from the outcome) were those that had been through the formal process of being registered blind or partially sighted, or received an assessment from the Blind Team. This process appeared to come closest to containing all the positive components discussed above and considered by respondents to constitute a 'proper' assessment. It consisted of a face to face meeting (sometimes more than one meeting) with a practitioner. People were given plenty of information in a variety of accessible formats before, during and after the face to face meeting about both the process and the outcome of the assessment or registration process. The process had a clearly defined and formalised structure. The basis for decisions about people's needs was fully explained, and there was a clear, explicit, formal system for challenging those decisions. In other words, the assessment procedures were explicit and formalised, and thus would, theoretically, be open to challenge using judicial-type processes.

Disabled people and their families recognised the following elements as characteristic of a full assessment: it took place face to face, with the practitioner, and where relevant, with other practitioners from involved agencies present; they were given sufficient notice and time to prepare themselves, or sufficient time and space within the assessment meeting to discuss their needs; they were given sufficient information about both the assessment process and outcome of the assessment to make informed choices about their needs and the relevant services, equipment and support; they were treated as a competent member of society by the practitioner; the process was explicit and formal and decisions made within were challengeable; and they were assessed by a practitioner who was willing to share information and act, where necessary as an advocate, who acted as a welfare broker illuminating the complex community care and wider welfare system, and who gave sound, pragmatic advice based on experience. This evidence suggests that the variation in assessment procedures, particularly those that allow practitioners to operate bureaucratic gatekeeping mechanisms to prevent disabled people accessing an assessment should be replaced by a common, formalised, explicit system of assessment that is clear, fair and open to challenge by disabled people and their families.

Who Should Carry Out Assessments?

There were several aspects of the variation in assessment procedures that had implications for the citizenship status of disabled people. The first was the identity of the person carrying out the assessment. As Ellis (1993) and others have pointed out, asking practitioners working at the front-line to square the conflicting community care policy objectives of limiting access to scarce resources and the professional objective of empowering (potential) service users within their daily practice is a difficult, almost impossible task. The evidence in this study shows that where there was insufficient managerial support for practitioners concerned with enabling disabled people to access a full assessment, thus protecting their civil and social rights, the 'deep normative core' of community care policy (i.e. rationing access to scarce resources) (Lewis and Glennerster, 1996) would take precedence in both the managerially and bureaucratically designed procedures practitioners used to decide who should gain access to assessments and services.

It is not only the fact that practitioners were (apart from in the Blind Team) employees of, and therefore accountable to, the local authorities that caused concern. It was also the way in which they used their professional status (usually as qualified social workers) as well as their necessarily enhanced knowledge of the systems and procedures in use to justify adopting what was referred to earlier in this book as a 'citizen-the-worker' approach to assessment. This meant that they considered themselves to be the experts not only in the procedures, eligibility criteria and assessment systems used by the local authority and their own individual teams, but also in defining what constituted a disabled or older person's needs, particularly doing what Cheetham (1993) characterises as the skilled job of separating out needs from desires, better than the disabled person was able to do themselves. Within the assessment arena such practitioners considered themselves to be the 'most competent' person, by reason of their professional training and status, to undertake such tasks.

However, two important points about the identity of the assessor and professional competence emerged from the data presented in this study. Firstly, the 'citizen-the-worker' approach was not adopted uniformly by all practitioners. It tended to flourish where there was explicit managerial support for the use of bureaucratic gatekeeping mechanisms to ration access to scarce resources by limiting the numbers of people accessing a full assessment. In other words, there was a correlation between the adoption of the 'deep normative core' of community care policy (rationing access to resources) as the driving value of assessment procedures and the constitution of the practitioner as the 'citizen-worker'. In teams where the 'deep normative core' of community care policy took lower precedence in assessment procedures it was much more common to find practitioners adopting a 'co-citizen' approach to assessment, where the expertise of the practitioner (in the procedures, and their knowledge about the availability of services) was matched by the disabled person's knowledge about their own needs. In other words, managerial support to adopt a 'co-citizen' approach to assessment could successfully overcome the drawbacks of having to implement the 'deep normative core' of rationing access to resources.

Secondly, there were aspects of the practitioners' competence and expertise that were valued by disabled people and their families, but these were not the skills at separating needs from desires valued by Cheetham (1993) and other defenders of the value of professional social workers as assessors. Disabled people and their families attached great importance to the role that practitioners played in guiding them through the complex community care system, and often the wider welfare state as well. The interviewees in this study were usually very clear and knowledgeable about their own needs and what they needed in order to be able to function as citizens, or 'competent members of society' engaging in 'minimally curtailed social participation'. They were less clear about how to access an assessment of those needs, or the range or availability of services, equipment and support that might meet those needs. This was where the practitioners enhanced expertise came into play and was valued by disabled people and their families. Many respondents pointed out how much they valued the practical assistance with negotiating the welfare system (including help with areas not considered to be 'core business' by some social services departments, such as social security and housing problems, which were nonetheless considered to be 'core needs' by the interviewees).

Practitioners who had personal experience of disability were particularly appreciated, as they understood the physical, attitudinal and social barriers faced by many of the respondents, and had experience that they were willing to share as 'co-citizens' with respondents. Although some of these experiences were based around sharing similar impairments and therefore centred on pragmatic issues such as the best equipment to use, even respondents whose practitioners had different impairments reported that the shared experience of disability - the social barriers experienced by those with impairments - also made the relationship with those practitioners qualitatively different to relationships with non-disabled practitioners. Such practitioners tended to adopt a 'co-citizenship' approach to assessments where the disabled person's knowledge of their own needs was accorded equal value with the practitioner's knowledge of assessment systems and the range and availability of services, equipment and support to meet those needs. Where they were given sufficient managerial support it was also possible, although less common, for non-disabled practitioners to adopt a similar 'co-citizenship' approach to assessment.

It might be that one characteristic element of a 'co-citizenship' approach to assessment was the build up of trust that took place between practitioners and applicants. The sharing of the experience of disability was obviously an important part of the development of that trusting relationship for many respondents. However, non-disabled practitioners who took the time to build up relationships with disabled people by allowing them the time and space within the assessment process to articulate their needs, and who did not behave as though their professional status made them more of an expert on those needs than the disabled person themselves, were much appreciated. It was just as important for the build up of trust that practitioners were honest about delays, resource restrictions, application procedures and the scarcity of services, rather than trying to persuade applicants that an assessment or particular service or piece of equipment was not needed.

Developing a 'Co-citizenship' Approach to Assessments: the Role of Social Services Departments

Both the concerns outlined above - the degree of formalisation of the assessment process, and the identity and skills of the person carrying out the assessment - suggest that the organisation and funding of assessments and the role of local authority-employed social workers within that process should be questioned. The evidence in this study suggests that the assessment process should be formalised, the criteria upon which decisions about who should access assessments and services made explicit and therefore open to scrutiny and challenge within a welfare rights context (making the right to an assessment a meaningful one upholdable in law). This leads to the conclusion that the degree of discretion that local authorities have in designing and implementing assessment procedures should be removed, particularly the degree in which they are able to implement and use bureaucratic gatekeeping mechanisms to deter or limit the number of applicants accessing a full community care assessment.

In effect this would reshape assessments as something closer to some of the spirit of the NHSCCA, particularly in making them needs-led, rather than service-led. However, there would still remain the problem of the identity of the assessor. Even if assessments were formalised and the criteria made explicit and challengeable, if social services departments retain the responsibility for carrying them out AND are the ones responsible for providing services and rationing access to scarce resources, the problems of 'squaring the circle' for frontline practitioners remain (Ellis, 1993). It would appear from the evidence in this study that better assessment practice is linked to removing at least some of the immediate pressures to ration access to resources from frontline practitioners. Those practitioners who received managerial support to do so were able to allow disabled people and their families the time and space to explore their needs, without necessarily making any bigger claims on resources or services than those who had undergone rushed assessments at a pace, venue and procedure dictated by the 'deep normative core' to ration access to resources.

However, concerns about the identity of the assessor were not limited to the fact that they were employed by the organisation responsible for providing and rationing access to services. As the discussion above highlighted, disabled people and their families valued practitioners who adopted a 'co-citizenship' approach to assessment (where the expertise that disabled people had about their own needs was balanced by the expertise that the assessor had about criteria, procedures and services) over those that adopted a 'citizen-the-worker' approach (where the practitioner was considered both the most competent to assess the disabled person's needs, and had all the relevant knowledge about criteria, procedures and services). They particularly valued it when practitioners adopted a pragmatic rather than professional approach to assessment. Rather than using their professional training to help disabled people discover their needs (when they were perfectly capable of doing this themselves), such practitioners often acted as welfare brokers, assisting people in making informed choices about the range of options available to help them meet their needs, where necessarily acting as advocates on behalf of disabled people and their families.

These findings would indicate that in order to protect and enhance the citizenship status of disabled people, the process of assessment needs to be formalised and to work at arms length from the process of allocating resources. Similarly, the work of welfare rights indicates that in order to be able to act as advocates, workers need a degree of independence from the organisation responsible for providing access to resources to meet needs (Alcock, 1989; Fimister, 1986). This leads to the conclusion that the function of assessment could perhaps be removed from social services departments altogether. Within the context of this study this had happened in one of the teams - the Blind Team - which had contracted from the local authority the formal process of registration and community care assessments for blind and partially sighted people. It is notable that respondents were, on the whole, much more satisfied with both the process and outcome of their assessments than those who had been assessed by local authority social services departments.

Some of the benefits reported by such respondents, such as easier access to assessments, good quality information about the process, clear and challengeable criteria and practitioners who used a pragmatic, 'co-citizenship' approach to assessment, were shared by respondents who had accessed assessments from local authority practitioners, particularly those in the Younger Person's Team and the Deaf Team. These latter teams also offered practitioners managerial support in the way assessment procedures operated to work at arms length from rationing decisions. In particular, the use of a 'co-citizenship' approach to assessment appears to be crucial, and made easier in all three teams by the way in which disabled practitioners worked alongside their non-disabled colleagues. The logical conclusion to these findings, in particular to the difficulties experienced by the other teams in using a 'co-citizenship' approach to assessment, indicates that an organisation run by disabled people themselves and driven by their aims and needs, rather than by the 'deep normative core' of community care policy of rationing access to resources, offers the best hope of delivering quality assessment practice that is both acceptable to practitioners and protects and enhances the citizenship status of disabled people.

One solution might be to contract out the 'new improved formalised' assessment process to organisations run by disabled people themselves rather than allowing local authority social services departments to carry on undertaking these responsibilities. This would enable assessors to act as pragmatic welfare brokers, assisting disabled people to find their way through the complex welfare and community care system, and where necessary acting as advocates on their behalf against local authorities who would retain the responsibility for rationing access to scarce welfare resources. The pressure to use a 'citizen-the-worker' approach to assessment would be much reduced, and where decisions needed to be challenged the ethos and practice of welfare rights work could be used to protect the civil and social rights of disabled citizens.

This may work well with younger disabled people or those with specific impairments, such as happened in the Blind Team (which was funded partly through the local authority and partly through a local branch of the Royal National Institute for the Blind, an independent charitable foundation). However, older disabled people in the UK have a less developed history of collective self-advocacy, although some key projects have overcome this (Barnes and Bennett-Emslie, 1995). The evidence in this study shows that individual articulate older disabled people could and did challenge practitioners successfully when they felt they have been unfairly treated by practitioners using a 'citizen-the-worker' approach to assessment, but it is difficult for individuals to challenge bureaucratic gatekeeping decisions because, by their nature, such decisions are implicit and informal. It is therefore even more crucial for the protection of older disabled people's citizenship status that the assessment process is formalised, laid open to challenge, and undertaken by practitioners who use a 'co-citizenship' approach. Perhaps the situation will change as the current generation of disability activists and advocates grows older and local authorities are collectively challenged to change their practice in the way that they have done with younger disabled people (Goodin and Gibson, 1997).

The key elements of using the assessment process to enhance, rather than threaten disabled people's citizenship status are therefore as follows: formalise the process and protect disabled people's civil right to access an assessment; make the criteria upon which decisions about need are made clear, explicit and challengeable; develop a welfare rights approach to assessment, enabling disabled people to challenge discretionary decisions made by practitioners; enable practitioners to develop and use a 'co-citizenship' approach to assessment; support practitioners to act as pragmatic welfare rights brokers and advocates rather than professional experts on need; and create a working distance between the role of rationing access to scarce resources and the welfare brokerage role of assessment. One way of achieving these changes would be to remove the assessment function from social workers employed by social services departments and contract it out to organisations run by disabled people themselves.

The skills needed by practitioners to use a 'co-citizenship' approach to assessment should not be underestimated. Within the context of this study, even where practitioners were given a certain degree of protection from having to act as frontline rationers and explicit managerial support to use the assessment as a true arena to negotiate needs using a 'co-citizen' approach, there were still occasions where it was difficult for practitioners to avoid the power imbalance that was inherent in the encounter given their enhanced knowledge of the criteria, procedures and services available. Even disabled practitioners in the Blind Team acted on occasion as though their professional status made them more qualified to judge a disabled person's level of risk than the disabled person themselves, even when this meant they were clearly acting against that person's wishes. Appropriate training and support will be needed to enable assessment practitioners, whatever their professional and employment status, to adopt a 'co-citizenship' approach at all times during the process and to allow the disabled person's wishes and self-perceived needs to guide their actions. Citizenship does entail participating in society in the way in which individuals chose (Doyal and Gough, 1991) and that will involve making choices that are sometimes unpalatable to practitioners, but should nevertheless (within limits) be respected by them. Anti-discriminatory practice, long held to be one of the core values of professional social work, should enable differences to flourish and be respected within the assessment process.

A 'co-citizenship' approach to assessment is therefore a significant challenge for welfare professionals to adopt. It goes beyond an understanding and implementation of a social model of disability and requires practitioners to critically examine and, where necessary, challenge their values and views about the role of their work. Nevertheless there were numerous examples within this study of practitioners using a co-citizenship approach to assessment that was valued by managers, disabled people and their families and practitioners themselves. The role of managerial support and ongoing training for practitioners is vital within the assessment process. This would be the case whether the present system of variable discretionary procedures being used by local authorities continued, or if a new form of formalised, explicit assessment procedure contracted out to organisations run by and for the interests of disabled people themselves were adopted.

Developing Citizen-Friendly Services

Of course, accessing an assessment as a welfare good is only really of value because it is the pathway to accessing the services, equipment and support that many disabled people and their families need in order to be able to participate fully in society as competent citizens. In this study, what social services departments would characterize as the process of 'care management' and what respondents would recognize as the outcome of an assessment was intrinsically bound up with the process of 'assessment'. The reason these encounters with practitioners were so crucial for respondents, and why the nature of them had such an effect on their citizenship status was due in a large part to the relationship between the assessment itself and the way in which respondents experienced the receipt of services, equipment and support. Any attention given to improving the process of assessment and encouraging a 'co-citizenship' approach to be developed and used must be matched by attention given to the relationship between the outcome of the process and disabled people's citizenship status. It is clear from the evidence presented in this study that there were several areas in which the delivery of services could act as a barrier to disabled people's ability to engage in 'minimally curtailed social participation'.

Control Over Services

The lack of control over the delivery of services experienced by many disabled people was a serious concern for them and their families. Services tended to be organised to meet the needs of service providers rather than users, and consequently disabled people often found they had little control over the quality or timing of services. They often found that services were inappropriate or insufficiently flexible to meet their needs, with the consequence that they experienced additional barriers to their social participation. Such services often led to disabled people and their families experiencing increased social exclusion and isolation. On the other hand, services which were timely, appropriate, flexible and delivered in such a way that they were controlled by disabled people themselves often had the effect of enhancing their citizenship status by enabling them to participate in society in the way that they chose, including fulfilling caring and other duties. Such services often led to disabled people and their families experiencing greater levels of social participation.

It is clear that wherever possible services need to be adaptable, flexible and responsive to disabled people's needs. It is also clear that for this to be the case, disabled people and their families need to be given much greater control over the delivery of services than is presently the norm. One possible way of doing this is through the extension of the current scheme of direct payments, where disabled people are given money to purchase their own support and services in a way that suits them, rather than receiving services designed and organised to meet the needs of service providers (Glendinning et al, 2000; Hasler et al, 1999; Kestenbaum, 1992; Zarb and Naidash, 1994).

Such schemes have been welcomed by disabled people in the UK as offering a solution to the failure of community care policy to empower disabled people (Morris, 1997) because of the conflicting objectives contained within the policy. Other commentators have warned against the dangers of 'commodifying care' and expressed concerns that such schemes rely on the labour of underpaid unqualified workers, usually women (Ungerson, 1995, 1997). There are some problems with this type of scheme, such as the underdevelopment of a proper 'market' in personal assistants and other service providers to enable direct payments users to exercise the options of choice and exit, the lack of training and career development for personal assistants, the underfunding of payments particularly to those with complex needs (including the lack of contribution to direct payments from the NHS), the low takeup of direct payments by local authorities, and the lack of support for disabled people in managing payments and staff

(Glendinning et al, 2000; Hasler et al, 1999).

However, there is evidence to suggest that people using direct payments schemes do so because it offers significant benefits over traditional services, particularly in the way in which services can be controlled and made flexible and responsive to needs by the disabled person themselves (Glendinning et al, 2000). One of the key problems with the implementation of direct payments from the perspective of those using them appears to be the same problems experienced by some of the respondents in this study: the dissonance in definitions of need between assessors who are acting as gatekeepers to scarce resources and disabled people themselves. Funding for direct payments seems to reflect traditional service patterns rather than being truly needs-led.

Notwithstanding the fact that many direct payments packages are underfunded, the freedom and control given to disabled users of such schemes to construct and alter their own service packages to meet their needs in ways which suit them rather than ways which reflect the needs of service provider organisations is encouraging. It shows that there can be significant scope for enabling disabled people to participate in society in ways that they chose through a system that involves an element of assessment and rationing access to scarce resources. Perhaps the most challenging aspect of these findings is that direct payments users have successfully moved the focus on needs away from a narrow focus on the physical needs associated with their impairments towards a more holistic approach, including encompassing within the process a focus on the need to fulfil certain citizenship obligations or duties, such as childcare, work, education and leisure activities. In other words, it appears that using direct payments rather than receiving traditional services enhances disabled people's social participation, protecting their citizenship status.

Extending the possibilities offered by direct payments schemes without unnecessarily adding to or duplicating the weaknesses in them and thereby limiting the advantages offered by such schemes over traditional care management would be a significant challenge for local authorities. It would entail fundamentally changing the way in which they approach needs assessment and allowing the process to be led by disabled people's perceptions of their needs, rather than relying on historical patterns of service provision. In some ways this would involve an extension of the 'co-citizenship' approach to assessment to include a 'co-citizenship' approach to service delivery. Within a 'co-citizenship' approach to assessment, disabled people are considered experts in and competent to assess their own needs. A 'co-citizenship' approach to service delivery would extend that competency to include the competency to design and manage their own service packages. To use terminology more familiar to social services departments, developing citizen-friendly services involves allowing disabled people as far as possible to act as their own care managers.

The Disabled Care Manager

The implications of the findings concerning the impact accessing assessments and the assessment process itself lead to the conclusion that the function of assessment should be formalised and carried out at arms length from the function of rationing access to resources. The implications of the failure of traditional patterns of delivering services to protect or enhance the social inclusion and therefore citizenship status of disabled people are no less far reaching. It is clear that the expertise of 'co-citizen' type practitioners in the criteria, procedures and service options available is needed within the assessment process. However, as discussed above, in order for disabled people's citizenship status to be protected and enhanced by the support and services they receive, it is vital that they have control over the delivery of those services.

Having control over services does entail making choices and taking responsibility for the results of those choices: in other words, it involves acting as a 'competent member of society'. It might also involve making choices that would be unpalatable to care managers in the traditional mode, including the choice to refuse 'suitable' services and spend money on alternatives. Allowing disabled people to act as their own care managers would involve practitioners giving up a great deal of their power to shape people's lives by the decisions about the supply of services, support and equipment made on their behalf. It would remove the paternalistic element of care management completely, and so many care managers and commentators would probably argue that it would make disabled people unnecessarily vulnerable and dependent. I would argue that the evidence from this study and from studies of users of direct payments who are effectively acting as their own care managers suggest that many disabled people would accept this risk as a trade-off for the benefits of increased control and options for social inclusion offered by such responsibility.

A New Citizenship Framework: the Challenge for the Welfare State and its Citizens

This study raises wider questions that are relevant to social policy about the relationship between individual citizens and the state, particularly concerning the way in which citizens gain access to, and the state acts as the rationer of, scarce welfare resources. Are our current forms of citizenship suited to the challenges which face the welfare state? What are the implications for citizens and the state of the framework of citizenship as adapted from work by Marshall (1992), Turner (1993a), Doyal and Gough (1991) amongst others and used within the context of this study?

Firstly, the debate about the distinction between civil and social rights is slightly misleading. As constituted within this book, civil rights are those rights which are upholdable within a judicial context, which is not strictly how Marshall envisaged them (Marshall, 1992). It might be more accurate to say that what have been referred to throughout this book as civil rights are more akin to what other commentators have called 'procedural rights' (Doyle and Harding, 1992). What they are called is less important than the issue of what they are, and how they can be protected. I maintain they are a key element in citizenship, and where they are threatened that threat impacts upon people's civil, procedural and social rights, and therefore upon they way in which they can participate in society, the degree of social exclusion they experience and whether or not they can act as and are treated as 'competent members of society'. Much of the debate on the future nature of the welfare state has focused on the outcome of its function: the range of welfare goods available, their cost and effectiveness (see for example Glennerster, 2000; Hills, 1990). I would argue that the issue of the process of welfare delivery, how people gain access to these services and the way in which agents of the state make decisions about people's needs should receive just as much attention.

Secondly, if we are to focus on the process of welfare delivery then the role of practitioners comes under much greater scrutiny. As was discussed previously, rationing is an emotive term (Klein et al, 1996) and practitioners themselves are often unhappy with it (see for example recent debates about the role of GPs within primary care groups rationing access to NHS resources). But however unpalatable, the truth remains that the role of professionals within the welfare state as it is presently constituted within the context of the UK (and most other similar welfare states) is to ration access to scare resources. Where this happens covertly practitioners are granted a great deal of largely discretionary and unchallengeable power to make decisions which significantly affect citizen's lives and can dramatically impact upon the level of social inclusion or exclusion that they experience. This can make individual citizens vulnerable to the excess power of the state, a situation that is constitutionally unacceptable. The only way to protect citizens against such possible power abuses by the agents of the state is to make practitioners' rationing decisions explicit and make practitioners accountable to citizens for them.

Finally, the implications of these arguments are that the relationship between individual citizens and the welfare state needs to change. At present it appears to be characterised by a system in which decisions about rationing scarce resources are taken by agents of the state on behalf of individual citizens with insufficient power residing in citizens to either be involved in such decisions or to challenge or overturn them. This is not an easy challenge to tackle. Schemes and pilots to encourage citizen participation in decisions about rationing (or 'deciding service priorities') abound within social services, the NHS and other areas of the welfare state. So far there is little evidence to suggest that they have had much impact on addressing the power imbalance in the relationship between individuals and the state, and very few of them focus on the power imbalance inherent in the process of welfare delivery. This also has implications for the role of individual citizens, who must be willing and able to take up the challenge of being involved in unpalatable decisions about service priorities and rationing, and treating practitioners as 'co-citizens' and calling them to account for their decisions. Adopting a new citizenship framework that protects the civil, procedural and social rights of citizens while preventing agents of the state acting in a paternalistic way will be a significant challenge for both individual citizens and practitioners, managers and policy makers. Critically examining the development of that framework is the challenge left to social policy commentators in the new century.

Bibliography

Alcock, P (1989) 'Why Citizenship and Welfare Rights Offer New Hope for Welfare in Britain', *Critical Social Policy*, 19:26; pp.32-43.

Alcock, P (1996) *Social Policy in Britain: Themes and issues*, Basingstoke, Macmillan.

Allen, I, Dalley, G and Leat, D (1992) *Monitoring Change in Social Services Departments*, London, Policy Studies Institute.

Arber, S and Ginn, J (1995) *Connecting Gender and Ageing*, Buckingham, Open University Press.

Audit Commission (1986) *Making a Reality of Community Care*, London, HMSO.

Audit Commission (1993) *Taking Care: Progress with care in the community*, London, HMSO.

Audit Commission (1996) *Balancing the Care Equation: Progress with community care*, London, HMSO.

Baldock, J and Ungerson, C (1991) 'What D'ya Want if You Don' Want Money? A feminist critique of "paid volunteering"', in M Maclean and D Groves (eds) *Women's Issues in Social Policy*, London, Routledge.

Baldock, J and Ungerson, C (1993) *Becoming Consumers of Community Care*, York, Joseph Rowntree Foundation.

Baldwin, S and Falkingham, J (1994) *Social Security and Social Change: New challenges to the Beveridge model*, Hemel Hempstead, Harvester Wheatsheaf.

Baldwin, S and Lunt, N (1996) *Charging Ahead: The development of local authority charging policies for community care*, Bristol, Policy Press.

Barbalet, JM (1988) *Citizenship: Rights, struggle and class inequality*, Milton Keynes, Open University Press.

Barbalet, JM (1993) *'Citizenship, Class Inequality and Resentment'*, in BS Turner (ed), *Citizenship and Social Theory*, London, Sage.

Barker, I and Peck, D (1987) *Power in Strange Places: User empowerment in mental health services*, London, Good Practices in Mental Health.

Barnes, C (1991) *Discrimination and Disabled People in Britain*, London, Hurst & Co.

Barnes, M (1997) *Care, Communities and Citizens*, London, Longman.

Barnes, M (1999) 'Users as Citizens: Collective action and the local governance of welfare', *Social Policy and Administration*, 33:1; pp 73-90.

Barnes, M and Bennett-Emslie, G (1995) *If They Would Listen: An evaluation of the Fife User Panels Project*, Edinburgh, Age Concern Scotland.

Barnes, M and Prior, D (1995) 'Spoilt for Choice: How consumerism can disempower public-service users', *Public Money and Management*, 15:3; pp.53-58.

Barnes, M, Prior, D and Thomas, N (1990) 'Social Services', in N Deakin and A Wright (eds), *Consuming Public Services*, London, Routledge.

Barnes, M and Walker, A (1996) 'Consumerism Versus Empowerment: A principles approach to the involvement of older service users', *Policy and Politics*, 24:4; pp.375-393.

Barry, N (1987) 'Understanding the Market', in M Loney and R Bocock (eds), *The State or the Market: Politics and welfare in contemporary Britain*, London, Sage.

Bell, L (1987) 'Survivors Speak Out: A national self-advocacy network', in I Barker and D Peck (eds) *Power in Strange Places: User empowerment in mental health services*, London, Good Practices in Mental Health.

Bennett, JT and Johnson, MH (1980) 'Tax Reduction Without Sacrifice: Private sector production of public services', *Public Finance Quarterly*, 8:4; pp.368-396.

Beresford, P and Croft, S (1993) *Citizen Involvement*, Basingstoke, Macmillan.

Bewley, C and Glendinning, C (1994) 'Representing the Views of Disabled People in Community Care Planning Disability', *Handicap and Society*, 9:3; pp.301-314.

Biehal, N, Fisher, M, Marsh, P and Sainsbury, E (1992) 'Rights and Social Work', in A Coote (ed), *The Welfare of Citizens*, London, Institute of Public Policy Research.

Biggs, S (1994) 'Failed Individualism in Community Care: An example from elder abuse', *Journal of Social Work Practice*, 8:2; pp.137-149.

Blackman, T (1999) 'Facing Up to Underfunding: Equity and retrenchment in community care', *Social Policy and Administration*, 32:2; pp.182-195.

Bock, G and James, S (1992) *Beyond Equality and Difference*, London, Routledge.

Booth, T and Booth, W (1994) *Parenting Under Pressure: Mothers and fathers with learning difficulties*, Buckingham, Open University Press.

Bornat, J, Pereira, C, Pilgrim, D and Williams, F (eds) (1993) *Community Care: A reader*, Basingstoke, Macmillan.

Bosanquet, N (1983) *After the New Right*, London, Heinemann.

Bosanquet, N and Propper, C (1991) 'Charting the Grey Economy in the 1990s', *Policy and Politics*, 9:4; pp.269-282.

Bradshaw, J and Gibbs, I (1988) *Public Support for Private Residential Care*, Aldershot, Avebury.

Braham, P, Rattansi, A and Skellington, R (1992) *Racism and Anti-racism*, London, Sage.

Braye, S and Preston-Shoot, M (1995) *Empowering Practice in Social Care*, Buckingham, Open University Press.

Brisenden, S (1985) *A Charter for Personal Care*, Hampshire, HCIL.

Brisenden, S (1989) *A Charter for Personal Care Progress*, 16, London, Disablement Income Group.

Brown, M (1972) *The Development of Local Authority Welfare Services from 1948-1965 under Part II of the National Assistance Act 1948, PhD thesis*, University of Manchester.

Bulmer, M and Rees, AM (eds) (1996) *Citizenship Today: The contemporary relevance of TH Marshall*, London, University College London Press.

Burkitt, B and Davey, AG (1984) *Radical Political Economy: An introduction to the alternative economics*, Brighton, Wheatsheaf Books.

Butler, J and Scott, JW (eds) (1992) *Feminists Theorize the Political*, London, Routledge.

Butterworth, E and Holman, R (eds) (1975) *Social Welfare in Modern Britain*, London, Fontana.

Bynoe, I (1996) *Beyond the Citizen's Charter: New directions for social rights*, London, Institute for Public Policy Research.

Cahill, M (1994) *The New Social Policy*, Oxford, Blackwell.

Cass, B (1994) 'Citizenship, Work and Welfare: The dilemma for Australian women', *Social Politics*, 1:1; pp.106-124.

Challis, D (1992) *The Community Care of Elderly People: Bringing together scarcity and choice, needs and costs*, PSSRU Discussion Paper #813, Canterbury, University of Kent.

Challis, D, Darton, R, Johnson, L, Stone, M and Traske, K (1995) *Care Management and Health Care of Older People: The Darlington Community Care Project*, Aldershot, Arena.

Cheetham, J (1993) 'Social Work and Community Care in the 1990s: Pitfalls and potentials', in R Page and J Baldock (eds) *Social Policy Review 5*, London, Social Policy Association.

Chetwynd, M and Ritchie, R in collaboration with Reith, L and Howard, M (1996), *The Cost of Care: The impact of charging policy on the lives of disabled people*, York, Joseph Rowntree Foundation.

Clarke, H, Dyer, S and Horwood, J (1998) *That Bit of Help: The high value of low level preventative services for older people*, Bristol, Policy Press.

Clarke, J and Newman, J (1997) *The Managerial State*, London, Sage.

Cooper, L, Coote, A, Davies, A and Jackson, C (1995) *Voices Off: Tackling the Democratic Deficit in Health*, London, Institute for Public Policy Research.

Coote, A (ed) (1992) *The Welfare of Citizens*, London, Institute of Public Policy Research.

Croft, S and Beresford, P (1990) *From Paternalism to Participation: Involving people in social services*, London, Open Services Project.

Culpitt, I (1992) *Welfare and Citizenship: Beyond the crisis of the welfare state?*, London, Sage.

Dahrendorf, R (1988) 'Citizenship and the Modern Social Conflict', in R Holme and M Elliott (eds), *The British Constitution 1688-1988*, Basingstoke, Macmillan.

Dahrendorf, R (1996) 'Citizenship and Social Class', in M Bulmer and AM Rees (eds), *Citizenship Today: The contemporary relevance of TH Marshall*, London, University College London Press.

Dalley, G (1988) *Ideologies of Caring: Rethinking community and collectivism*, Basingstoke, Macmillan.

Daniels, AK (1967) 'The Low-caste Stranger in Social Research' in G Sjoberg (ed) *Ethics, Politics and Social Research*, Cambridge MA, Schenkman.

Davis, A, Ellis, K and Rummery, K (1997) *Access to Assessment: perspectives of practitioners, disabled people and carers*, Policy Press, Bristol.

Deakin, N and Wright, A (eds) (1990) *Consuming Public Services*, London, Routledge.

Department of Health (1989) *Caring for People: Community care in the next decade and beyond*, London, HMSO.

Department of Health (1990) *Community Care in the Next Decade and Beyond*, London, HMSO.

Department of Health (1993) *Implementing Community Care: Population needs assessment, good practice guidelines*, London, Department of Health.

Department of Health (1999) *Community Care (Direct Payments) Act 1996: Draft policy and practice guidance*, Consultation paper, London, Department of Health.

Department of Health and Social Security (1981) *Growing Older*, London, HMSO.

Dietz, M (1987) *Context Is All: Feminism and theories of citizenship*, Daedalus, 116:4; pp.1-24.

Doyal, L and Gough, I (1991) *A Theory of Human Need*, Basingstoke, Macmillan.

Doyle, N and Harding, T (1992) 'Community Care: Applying procedural fairness', in A Coote (ed), *The Welfare of Citizens*, London, Institute of Public Policy Research.

Drewett, AY (1999) 'Social Rights and Disability: The language of "rights" in community care policies', *Disability and Society*, 14:1; pp.115-128.

Driedger, D (1989) *The Last Civil Rights Movement: Disabled People's International*, London, Hurst.

Drucker, P (1969) 'The Sickness of Government', *The Public Interest*, 14; pp.3-23.

Einhorn, B (1993) *Cinderella Goes to Market*, London, Verso.

Ellis, K (1993) *Squaring the Circle: User and carer participation in needs assessment*, York, Joseph Rowntree Foundation.

Ellis, K, Davis, A and Rummery, K (1999) 'Needs Assessment, "street-level bureaucracy" and the new community care', *Social Policy and Administration*,

Esping-Anderson, G (1990) *The Three Worlds of Welfare Capitalism*, Oxford, Blackwell.

Fielding, N (1993) 'Ethnography', in N Gilbert, (ed), *Researching Social Life*, London, Sage.

Fimister, G (1986) *Welfare Rights Work in Social Services*, Basingstoke, Macmillan.

Finch, J (1985) 'Work, the Family and the Home: A more egalitarian future', *International Journal of Social Economics*, 12:1; pp.26-35.

Finch, J (1989) *Family Obligations and Social Change*, Cambridge, Polity Press.

Finch, J and Groves, D (1980) 'Community Care and the Family: A case for equal opportunities?', *Journal of Social Policy*, 9:4; pp.487-571.

Finch, J and Groves, D (eds) (1983) *A Labour of Love: Women, work and caring*, London, Routledge and Kegan Paul.

Fraser, N (1989) 'Talking About Needs: Interpretive contests as political conflicts in welfare-state societies', *Ethics*, 99:2; pp.291-313.

Friedman, M (1962) *Capitalism and Freedom*, Chicago, University of Chicago Press.

Friedman, KA (1981) *Legitimation of Social Rights and the Western Welfare State: A Weberian perspective*, Chapel Hill, University of North Carolina Press.

Gilbert, N (ed) (1993) *Researching Social Life*, London, Sage.

Glaser, BG and Strauss, AL (1967) *The Discovery of Grounded Theory*, Chicago, Aldine.

Glennerster, H (2000) *Paying for Welfare: Towards 2000*, Hemel Hempstead, Harvester Wheatsheaf.

Glendinning, C (1983) *Unshared Care*, London, Routledge and Kegan Paul.

Glendinning, C (1991) 'Losing Ground: Social policy and disabled people in Britain 1980-90, *Disability, Handicap and Society*, 6:1; pp.3-19.

Glendinning, C (1992) *The Costs of Informal Care: Looking inside the household*, London, HMSO.

Glendinning, C (1993) 'Residualism vs Rights: Social policy and disabled people', in N Manning and R Page (eds), *Social Policy Review 4*, Canterbury, Social Policy Association.

Glendinning, C, Halliwell, S, Jacobs, S, Rummery, K and Tyrer, J (2000) *Buying Independence: Using direct payments to integrate health and social services*, Bristol, Policy Press.

Glendinning, C, Halliwell, S, Jacobs, S, Rummery K and Tyrer J (2000a) 'Bridging the Gap: Using direct payments to purchase integrated care', *Health and Social Care in the Community*, Vol.8, No.3: pp.192-201.

Glendinning, C and Millar, J (eds) (1992) *Women and Poverty in Britain: the 1990s*, Hemel Hempstead, Harvester Wheatsheaf.

Goffman, E (1961) *Asylums*, Harmondsworth, Penguin.

Goodin, RE and Gibson, D (1997) 'Rights, Young and Old', *Oxford Journal of Legal Studies*, 17; pp.185-203.

Goodin, RE and Le Grand, J (1987) *Not Only the Poor: The middle classes and the welfare state*, London, Allen and Unwin.

Graham, H (1983) 'Caring: A labour of love', in J Finch and D Groves (eds), *A Labour of Love: Women, work and caring*, London, Routledge and Kegan Paul.

Green, H (1988) *Informal Carers: General Household Survey 1985*, London, HMSO.

Gronbjerg, KA (1983) 'Private Welfare: Its future in the welfare state', *American Behavioral Scientist*, 26:6; pp.773-793.

Griffiths, R (1988) *Community Care: Agenda for Action*, London, HMSO.

Hantrais, L and Mangen, S (1994) *Family Policy and the Welfare of Women*, Loughborough, Cross-National Research Group.

Hardy, B, Young, R and Wistow, G (1999) 'Dimensions of Choice in the Assessment and Care Management Process: The views of older people, carers and care managers', *Health and Social Care in the Community*, 7:6; pp.483-491.

Hasler, F, Campbell, J and Zarb, G (1999) *Direct Routes to Independence*, London, NCIL and Policy Studies Institute.

Hayek, FA (1960) *The Constitution of Liberty*, Chicago, University of Chicago Press.

Hills, J (ed) (1990) *The State of Welfare: The welfare state in Britain since 1974*, Oxford, Oxford University Press.

Hills, J (1993) *The Future of Welfare*, York, Joseph Rowntree Foundation.

Hernes, H (1987) *Welfare State and Woman Power*, Oslo, Norwegian University Press.

Holme, R and Elliott, M (eds) (1998) *The British Constitution 1688-1988*, Basingstoke, Macmillan.

hooks, b (1982) *Ain't I a Woman?*, London, Pluto.

Hooyman, NR and Gonyea, J (1995) *Feminist Perspectives on Family Care: Policies for gender justice*, Thousand Oaks CA, Sage.

Hoyes, L, Jeffers, S, Lart, R, Means, R and Taylor, M (1993) *User Empowerment and the Reform of Community Care: An interim assessment*, Bristol, School for Advanced Urban Studies.

Huby, M and Dix, G (1992) *Evaluating the Social Fund*, London, Department of Social Security Research Report #9, HMSO.

Ignatieff, M (1984) *The Needs of Strangers*, London, Chatto and Windus.

Ignatieff, M (1989) 'Citizenship and Moral Narcissism', *The Political Quarterly*, 60:1; pp.63-74.

Institute of Housing (1990) *Housing Allocations: Report of a survey of Local Authorities in England and Wales*, Coventry, Institute of Housing.

John, P (1998) *Analysing Public Policy*, London, Pinter.

Joshi, H (1992) 'The Cost of Caring', in C Glendinning and J Millar (eds), *Women and Poverty in Britain: the 1990s*, Hemel Hempstead, Harvester Wheatsheaf.

Kestenbaum, A (1992) *Cash for Care: A report on the experiences of Independent Living Fund clients*, Nottingham, Independent Living Fund.

Kitzinger, C (1987) *The Social Construction of Lesbianism*, London, Sage.

Klein, R, Day, P and Redmayne, S (1996) *Managing Scarcity: Priority setting and rationing in the National Health Service*, Buckingham, Open University Press.

Laing, W (1993) *Financing Long-term Care: The critical debate*, London, Age Concern.

Lane, RE (1987) 'Market Justice, Political Justice', *Evaluation Studies Review Annual*,12; pp.343-362.

LeGrand, J (1982) *The Strategy of Equality*, London, George Allen and Unwin.

LeGrand, J and Bartlett, W (eds) (1993) *Quasi-Markets and Social Policy*, London, Macmillan.

LeGrand, J and Robinson R (1984) *The Economics of Social Problems: The market versus the welfare state*, London, Macmillan.

Lewis, J and Glennerster, H (1996) *Implementing the New Community Care*, Buckingham, Open University Press.

Lewis, J and Meredith, B (1988) *Daughters Who Care: Daughters caring for mothers at home*, London, Routledge and Kegan Paul.

Lipsky, M (1980) *Street Level Bureaucracy: Dilemmas of the individual in public services*, New York, Russell Sage Foundation.

Lister, R (1990) *The Exclusive Society: Citizenship and the Poor*, London, Child Poverty Action Group.

Lister, R (1995) 'Dilemmas in Engendering Citizenship', *Economy and Society*, 24:1; pp.1-38.

Lister, R (1997) *Citizenship: Feminist perspectives*, Basingstoke, Macmillan.

Lofland, J (1971) *Analysing Social Settings*, Belmont CA, Wadsworth.

Lofland, J and Lofland, LH (1984) *Analysing Social Settings*, Belmont CA, Wadsworth.

Loney, M and Bocock, R (eds) (1987) *The State or the Market: Politics and welfare in contemporary Britain*, London, Sage.

Lowther, C and Williamson, J (1996) 'Old People and Their Relatives', *Lancet*, 31 December: p.1460.

Maclean, M and Groves, D (eds) (1991) *Women's Issues in Social Policy*, London, Routledge.

Mackintosh, S, Means, R and Leather, P (1990) *Housing in Later Life*, SAUS Study #4, Bristol, School for Advanced Urban Studies.

Makkai, T (1994) 'Social Policy and Gender in Eastern Europe', in D Sainsbury (ed), *Gendering Welfare States*, London, Sage.

Mama, A (1992) 'Black Women and the British State', in P Braham, A Rattansi and R Skellington (eds), *Racism and Anti-racism*, London, Sage.

Mandelstam, M and Schwer, B (1995) *Community Care Practice and the Law*, London, Jessica Kingsley.

Manning, N and Page, R (eds) (1993) *Social Policy Review 4*, Canterbury, Social Policy Association.

Marshall, TH (1992) 'Citizenship and Social Class', in TM Marshall and T Bottomore, *Citizenship and Social Class*, London, Pluto.

Marshall, TH and Bottomore, T (1992) *Citizenship and Social Class*, London, Pluto.

McLaughlin, E and Glendinning, C (1994) 'Paying for Care in Europe: Is there a feminist approach?', in L Hantrais and S Mangen (eds), *Family Policy and the Welfare of Women*, Loughborough, Cross-National Research Group.

Meacher, M (1972) *Taken for a Ride*, London, Longmann.

Mead, L (1986) *Beyond Entitlement: The social obligations of citizenship*, New York, The Free Press.

Mead, LM (1997) 'Citizenship and Social Policy: TH Marshall and poverty', *Social Philosophy and Policy*, 14:2; pp.197-230.

Means, R (1986) 'The Development of Social Services for Elderly People: Historical perspectives', in C Phillipson and A Walker (eds), *Ageing and Social Policy: A critical assessment*, Aldershot, Gower.

Means, R and Smith, R (1994) *Community Care: Policy and Practice*, London, Macmillan.

Ministry of Health, (1957) *Local Authority Services for the Chronic Sick and Infirm*, Circular 14/57, London, HMSO.

Morris, J (1991) *Pride Against Prejudice*, London, Women's Press.

Morris, J (1992) 'Personal and Political: A feminist perspective in researching physical disability', *Disability, Handicap and Society*, 7:2.

Morris, J (1993a) *Community Care or Independent Living?*, York, Joseph Rowntree Foundation.

Morris, J (1993b) *Independent Lives: Community Care and Disabled People*, Basingstoke, Macmillan.

Morris, J (ed) (1996) *Encounters with Strangers: Feminism and disability*, London, Women's Press.

Morris, J (1997) 'Care or Empowerment: A disability rights perspective', *Social Policy and Administration*, 31:1; pp.54-60.

Mouffe, C (1992) 'Feminism, Citizenship and Democratic Politics', in J Butler and JW Scott (eds), *Feminists Theorize the Political*, London, Routledge.

Murray, C (1990) *The Emerging British Underclass*, London, The IEA Health and Welfare Unit.

Myers, F and Macdonald, C (1996) 'Power to the People? Involving users and carers in needs assessment and care planning - views from the practitioner', *Health and Social Care in the Community*, 4:2; pp.86-96.

NHSME (1992) *Local Voices: The views of local people in purchasing for health*, London, Department of Health.

Oliver, M (1990) *The Politics of Disablement*, Basingstoke, Macmillan.

Oliver, M and Barnes, C (1993) 'Discrimination, Disability and Welfare: From needs to rights', in J Swain, V Finkelstein, S French and M Oliver (eds), *Disabling Barriers - Enabling Environments*, Milton Keynes, Open University/Sage.

Page, R and Baldock, J (eds) (1993) *Social Policy Review 5*, London, Social Policy Association.

Parker, G (1993) *With This Body: Caring and disability in marriage*, Buckingham, Open University Press.

Parker, R (1975) 'Social Administration and Scarcity', in E Butterworth and R Holman (eds), *Social Welfare in Modern Britain*, London, Fontana.

Pateman, C (1992) 'Equality, Difference, Subordination: The politics of motherhood and women's citizenship', in G Bock and S James (eds) *Beyond Equality and Difference*, London, Routledge.

Phillipson, C and Walker, A (eds) (1986) *Ageing and Social Policy: A critical assessment*, Aldershot, Gower.

Plant, R (1988) *Citizenship, Rights and Socialism*, London, Fabian Society.

Plant, R (1990) 'Citizenship and Rights', in R Plant and N Barry (eds), *Citizenship and Rights in Thatcher's Britain: Two views*, London, IEA Health and Welfare Unit.

Plant R (1992) 'Citizenship, Rights and Welfare' in A Coote (ed), *The Welfare of Citizens*, London, Institute of Public Policy Research.

Plant, R and Barry, N (1990) *Citizenship and Rights in Thatcher's Britain: Two views*, London, IEA Health and Welfare Unit.

Platt, J (1981) 'Evidence and Proof in Documentary Research', *Sociological Review*, 29:1; pp.31-66.

Pratt, HJ (1993) *Gray Agendas: Interest groups and public pensions in Canada, Britain and the United States*, Michigan, University of Michigan Press.

Qureshi, H, Patmore, C, Nicholas, E and Bamford, C, (1998) *Overview: Outcomes of Social Care for Older People and Carers*, York, SPRU and University of York.

Rees, AM (1996) 'TH Marshall and the Progress of Citizenship', in M Bulmer and AM Rees (eds), *Citizenship Today: The contemporary relevance of TH Marshall*, London, University College London Press.

Richards, E (1996) *Estimating the Costs of Long Term Care*, London, Institute of Public Policy Research.

Richards, M (1996) *Community Care for Older People: Rights, remedies and finances*, Bristol, Jordans.

Roche, M (1992) *Rethinking Citizenship*, Cambridge, Polity Press.

Rogers, A, Lacey, R and Pilgrim, D (1993) *Experiencing Psychiatry*, London, Macmillan.

Rogers, A and Pilgrim, D (1989) 'Mental Health and Citizenship', *Critical Social Policy*, 9:26; pp.44-55.

Rummery, K (2000) 'A Citizenship and Social Exclusion Issue? Access to health and social care for older people under New Labour', presented at the *Social Policy Association Annual Conference*, University of Surrey at Roehampton, July 2000.

Rummery, K, Ellis, K and Davis, A (1999) 'Negotiating Access to Assessments: Perspectives of front-line workers, disabled people and carers', *Health and Social Care in the Community*, 7:4; pp.296-300.

Rummery, K and Glendinning, C (1999) 'Negotiating Needs, Access and Gatekeeping: Developments in health and community care policies in the UK and the rights of disabled and older citizens', *Critical Social Policy*, 19:3; pp.335-351.

Rummery, K and Glendinning, C (2000) 'Access to Services as a Civil and Social Rights Issue: The role of welfare professionals in regulating access to and commissioning services for disabled and older people under New Labour', *Social Policy and Administration*, 34:5; pp.529-551.

Sainsbury, D (ed) (1994) *Gendering Welfare States*, London, Sage.

Salter, B (1994) 'The Politics of Community Care: Social rights and welfare limits', *Policy and Politics*, 22:2; pp.119-131.

Sheppard, M (1995) *Care Management and the New Social Work: A critical analysis*, London, Whiting and Birch.

Sjoberg, G (ed) (1967) *Ethics, Politics and Social Research*, Cambridge MA, Schenkman.

Spicker, P (1993) *Poverty and Social Security: Concepts and principles*, London, Routledge.

SSI/SSWG (1991) *Care Management and Assessment: A manager's guide*, London, HMSO.

Stevenson, O and Parsloe, P (1993) *Community Care and Empowerment*, York, Joseph Rowntree Foundation.

Stuart, O (1993) 'Double Oppression: An appropriate starting point?', in J Swain, V Finkelstein, S French and M Oliver (eds), *Disabling Barriers - Enabling Environments*, Milton Keynes, Open University/Sage.

Swain, J, Finkelstein, V, French, S and Oliver, M (eds) (1993) *Disabling Barriers - Enabling Environments*, Milton Keynes, Open University/Sage.

Taylor-Gooby, P (1985) 'Pleasing Any of the People, Some of the Time: Perceptions of redistribution and attitudes to welfare', *Government and Opposition*, 20:3; pp.396-406.

Thompson, A (1949) 'Problems of Ageing and Chronic Sickness', *British Medical Journal*, 30 July, pp.250-251.

Thompson, N (1993) *Anti-discriminatory Practice*, London, Macmillan.

Tinker, A (1996) *Older People in Modern Society*, Longman, London.

Townsend, P (1962) *The Last Refuge*, London, Routledge.

Townsend, P (1963) *The Family Life of Old People*, Harmondsworth, Penguin.

Townsend, P (1979) *Poverty in the United Kingdom*, Harmondsworth, Penguin.

Tulle-Winton, E (1995) 'Do You Remember Your Social Worker? Identification and recall problems in user surveys', in Wilson, G (ed) *Community Care: Asking the users*, London, Chapman and Hall.

Turner, BS (1986) *Citizenship and Capitalism: The debate over reformism*, London, Allen and Unwin.

Turner, BS (1990) 'Outline of a Theory of Citizenship', *Sociology*, 24:2; pp.189-217.

Turner, BS (ed) (1993) *Citizenship and Social Theory*, London, Sage.

Turner, BS (1993a) 'Contemporary Problems in the Theory of Citizenship', in BS Turner (ed), *Citizenship and Social Theory*, London, Sage.

Turner, BS (1993b) 'Outline of a Theory of Human Rights', in BS Turner (ed), *Citizenship and Social Theory*, London, Sage.

Twigg, J (1997) 'Bathing and the Politics of Care', *Social Policy and Administration*, 31:1, pp.61-72.

Ungerson, C (1992) 'Payment for Caring: Mapping a territory?' paper given at Social Policy Association Annual Conference, July, University of Nottingham.

Ungerson, C (1993) 'Caring and Citizenship: A complex relationship', in J Bornat et al (eds), *Community Care: A reader*, Basingstoke, Macmillan.

Ungerson, C (1995) 'Gender, Cash and Informal Care: European perspectives and dilemmas', *Journal of Social Policy*, 24:1; pp.31-52.

Ungerson, C (1997) 'Social Politics and the Commodification of Care', *Social Politics*, 4:3; pp.362-381.

UPIAS (1976) *Fundamental Principles of Disability, Union of Physically Impaired People Against Segregation*, London.

Walby, S (1994) 'Is Citizenship Gendered?', *Sociology*, 28:2; pp.379-395.

Walker, A and Warren, L (1996) *Changing Services for Older People*, Buckingham, Open University Press.

Walmsley, J (1993) '"Talking to Top People": Some issues relating to the citizenship of people with learning difficulties', in J Swain, V Finkelstein, S French and M Oliver (eds), *Disabling Barriers - Enabling Environments*, Milton Keynes, Open University/Sage.

Walmsley, J (1993a) 'Contradictions in Caring: Reciprocity and inter-dependence', *Disability, Handicap and Society*, 8:2; pp.129-141.

Walsh, K (1995) *Public Services and Market Mechanisms*, Basingstoke, Macmillan.

Weddell, K (1986) 'Privatising Social Services in the USA', *Social Policy and Administration*, 20:1; pp.14-27.

Wertheimer, A (1993) 'User Participation in Community Care: The challenge for services', in V Williamson (ed), *Users First: The real challenge for community care*, University of Brighton, Brighton.

Williamson, V (ed) (1993) *Users First: The real challenge for community care*, University of Brighton, Brighton.

Wilson, G (ed) (1995) *Community Care: Asking the users*, London, Chapman and Hall.

Wistow, G and Barnes, M (1995) 'User Involvement in Community Care: Origins, purposes and applications', *Public Administration*, 71:3; pp.279-299.

Wistow, G, Knapp, M, Hardy, B, Forder, J, Kendall, J and Manning, R (1996) *Social Care Markets: Progress and prospects*, Buckingham, Open University Press.

Williams, F (1989) *Social Policy: A critical introduction*, Cambridge, Polity Press.

Williams, GH (1991) 'Disablement and the Ideological Crisis in Health Care', *Social Science and Medicine*, 33:4; pp.517-524.

Yin, R (1984) *Case Study Research*, Beverly Hills CA, Sage.

Zarb, G and Naidash, P (1994) *Cashing In on Independence: Comparing the costs and benefits of cash and services*, London, British Council of Organisations of Disabled People.

Index